A Place of
MIRACLES

*The Story of a Children's Hospital in Kabul
and the People Whose Lives Have Been Changed by It*

To All Rose

Best regards,

Lee Hilling

10/8/11

D1114056

LEE HILLING

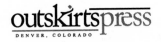
DENVER, COLORADO

A Place of Miracles
The Story of a Children's Hospital in Kabul and the People Whose Lives Have Been Changed by It

Contact info:
  Lee Hilling
  8326 North Brook Lane
  Bethesda, MD 20814
  301-654-1090
  LNHilling@verizon.net

Cover Image by Jean-Francois Mousseau

Outskirts Press, Inc.
http://www.outskirtspress.com

ISBN: 978-1-4787-4691-1

Library of Congress Control Number: 2014922642

Outskirts Press and the "OP" logo are trademarks belonging to Outskirts Press, Inc.

PRINTED IN THE UNITED STATES OF AMERICA

This book is dedicated to the marvelous staff at FMIC. They inspire and energize me. It is my honor to work with them in pursuit of their splendid mission.

TABLE OF CONTENTS

PROLOGUE: NEHA

WEBSTER'S DICTIONARY DEFINES a miracle as "an extraordinary event manifesting divine intervention in human affairs, an unusual event, thing, or accomplishment: wonder, marvel". There is a place where miracles happen, where one would not normally expect them: it's in Kabul, Afghanistan, at a place called the French Medical Institute for Children.

Gul Agha and his wife, Fazila, were desperate to save the lives of their precious new babies. Fazila had given birth to twin daughters only seven months into her pregnancy. Gul Agha got a call at work that Fazila was feeling ill and needed to see a doctor. He rushed her to a public hospital where the doctors decided a C-Section should be performed. One twin weighed 3 pounds 8 ounces at birth and the other just 1 pound 15 ounces. The hospital was unable to provide life-saving care to them. It had no facilities or staff to care for such tiny infants.

Gul Agha frantically searched all around Kabul trying to find a hospital that could care for the babies. A doctor at a private hospital told him she wouldn't admit them because she couldn't do anything for them. At a public hospital, another doctor refused to admit them because she didn't want to "damage the hospital's record at the end of the month," meaning, Gul Agha said, "they would die and she didn't want the bad statistic counted against her hospital." One of Kabul's largest public mother and child hospitals agreed to put the babies in an incubator for one night, but not for longer than that. It seemed only a miracle could save them. Finally, Gul Agha found his way to the French Medical Institute for Children, known locally as FMIC, and he was told the infants would be admitted and cared for there.

At FMIC, the tiny twins were admitted to the intensive care unit. It is the most advanced in Afghanistan and the only one in which the doctors and nurses can provide life-saving care for neonates – premature infants. It is a place of last resort for nearly all of its occupants. No other good choice exists for them. Under any circumstances, hospital intensive care units are places of awe. The most heart-rending ones are those that care for children and tiny infants. In the intensive care unit at FMIC the interplay of human drama and technology is gripping. Tubes, hoses, chords, electrodes, and needles protrude from, attach to, and poke into little bodies that are barely visible amidst all the paraphernalia. Anxious parents hover at their beloved children's sides, watching every act of nurses and doctors with a mix of desperation and hope. Hushed sounds – muted voices, hissing, clicking, and beeping – create an eerie, mystical aura. The families whose children are in the unit have an almost religious trust that miracles will happen and that their precious young lives will be saved.

At admission, the larger of the twins was diagnosed as having respiratory distress syndrome, a condition common in premature infants. She had also developed sepsis, a systemic infection which was life threatening in its own right. After admission, she developed a further complication in which blood clots formed throughout her body's small blood vessels. These combined conditions resulted in her death within three days. Now Gul Agha and Fazila were even more desperate for the remaining twin, Neha – the tiniest one – to survive.

Neha's weight dropped to 1 pound 12 ounces in her first few days in the hospital. Slowly, she responded to care and began to recover. She remained at FMIC for seventy-one days. She was discharged with the expectation that she would have a normal life. She was the smallest infant to ever be treated and survive in Afghanistan.

Dr. Amena Shaheer, the Afghan anesthetist who oversees the intensive care unit, said there was no place she could have survived in the country except at FMIC. "Some other hospitals have incubators, but they don't have the quality of facilities and of doctors and nurses that we do. Neha would have had no chance of survival if this hospital didn't exist,."

The total charge for Neha's care was US$6,839.00. Her family paid US$1,225.00, and the remaining US$5,614.00 was covered by the hospital's patient welfare program.

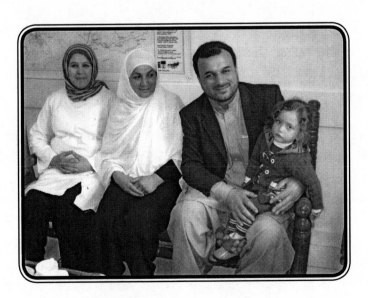

Neha with her parents and Dr. Amena

International combat forces and development agencies spent billions of dollars in Afghanistan in the years before and after FMIC's inauguration. Hospitals and clinics were built, but in some cases they were of such poor quality they were useless. In other cases, patients, doctors, and nurses – fearing Taliban retribution – were afraid to use them. Corruption was rampant. Sound oversight of contractors was often absent and the quality of completed projects was poor.

Back home, in the countries funding those initiatives, it seemed nothing done in Afghanistan had a good outcome. The Taliban was a re-emerging force and the prospect for outright victory or a negotiated settlement (at least one that would protect the interests of all Afghan citizens) looked increasingly unlikely.

Speaking at The Hague in 2009, then Secretary of State Hillary Rodham Clinton said that the billions of dollars spent in U.S. aid to Afghanistan over the past seven years were largely wasted and she called the amount of money spent without results "heartbreaking." In subsequent years, auditors found the situation unimproved.

FMIC is one of Afghanistan's most remarkable success stories. It has enabled children's lives to be saved that would otherwise have been lost, and it has enabled repair of children's disabilities and improvement to their quality of life. The partners creating FMIC have made an extraordinary contribution to increasing the capacity of Afghan doctors, nurses, allied health professionals, and management and support staff. FMIC has been a catalyst to enable Afghan health professionals to discover that they can perform at levels consistent with international standards and that they can interact with learned professionals from around the world.

Secretary of State Clinton may be correct that the amount of money spent in Afghanistan without results is "heartbreaking," but the investments in FMIC have achieved extraordinary results. My involvement with it has been one of the most uplifting experiences of my life. The story about FMIC is a story about miracles. It is a story about people who have succeeded and survived against overwhelming obstacles and odds, and it is a story about an institution that is the enabling catalyst for lives to be changed and dreams to be realized.

HOW WOULD YOU LIKE TO GO TO AFGHANISTAN?

The caller asked, "Lee, how would you like to go to Afghanistan?" I had never been to Afghanistan. About five seconds passed before I said, "Sure, why not."

The caller was the director of hospitals at Aiglemont, the site of the Aga Khan Development Network (AKDN) secretariat, or headquarters, in France. It was the same position I had held a few years earlier.

Having already accepted the invitation, it occurred to me that perhaps I should inquire why I was being asked to go to Afghanistan.

"A French non-governmental organization called La Chaîne de l'Espoir is constructing a children's hospital in Kabul," I was told. "They've approached the AKDN and asked us to assist them in running it."

"And what would you like me to do?"

"Lee, you know the AKDN doesn't have a history of working in partnerships. This would be very different from anything we have ever done. We'd like you to go there to assess the situation and make a recommendation back to us as soon as possible."

1

"And what would *as soon as possible* be?" I asked, thinking a little more about what I was getting myself into. My wife Pat and I were packed and ready to depart on an important trip from our home in Soddy-Daisy, Tennessee, near Chattanooga. We were going to the Outer Banks of North Carolina for our family's first ever reunion. Our kids and grandkids were traveling there from Massachusetts, Maryland, and Tennessee. We'd been planning this event for a long time. It hadn't been easy to find a time convenient for everybody.

"If you agree, we'd like you to go to Kabul as soon as possible and we'd like to get your report within a couple of months."

That was the beginning of my involvement with FMIC. It was June 2004. While the rest of my family was at the beach and lounging in the hot tub, I was getting my visa and airline tickets for my first trip to Afghanistan.

Afghanistan wasn't exactly a tourist destination in 2004. Three years earlier, on September 11, 2001, members of Al-Qaida, the Islamic terrorist organization led by Osama bin Laden, hijacked four American airliners. They crashed one into the Pentagon and two others into the World Trade Center towers. The fourth one, likely destined for either the U.S. Capitol or the White House, was commandeered by its brave passengers and crashed in a rural Pennsylvania meadow. At my home in Tennessee, I watched the scenes on television with disbelief and horror – over and over again.

America's immediate military response was directed toward Afghanistan. Within two weeks after the attacks, U.S. intelligence and special operations forces were on the ground there.

Within a month, *Operation Enduring Freedom* was begun. U.S.-led coalition airstrikes were launched with the goal of destroying Al-Qaida terrorist training camps and military installations operated by the Taliban, Al-Qaida's hosts in Afghanistan. By the end of the year, Osama bin Laden was on the run, the Taliban regime was toppled, and the Hamid Karzai government was installed.

My road to Kabul wasn't a straight line, but perhaps it was inevitable. My life and career up to that point hadn't been exactly straightforward and the invitation for me to go there wasn't a random event. I had a long history working with the AKDN.

I eagerly left life on the farm in Ohio and joined the U.S. Navy when I was just seventeen. My fascination with foreign places began with my first overseas assignment in Okinawa. When my ship docked in the port of Naha, the island had just experienced one of its frequent afternoon showers. Everything was as hot and steamy as a sauna. The heat and moisture added a musty quality and accentuated all the smells that were so alien to my nose. Discordant oriental music was blaring from speakers on the streets. I was swept away by the strange sights, sounds, and smells of the most exotic place I had ever seen. For a farm boy from Ohio it was like walking on the moon. For better or worse, I was hooked.

My next opportunity to travel abroad didn't come until 1966, when I was assigned to Vietnam as the administrator of a team of Navy doctors and hospital corpsmen caring for a civilian population in Chau Doc Province. Chau Doc was located on the Cambodian border in the Mekong Delta. Our team was a noncombatant component of a U.S. strategy intended to "win the hearts and minds" of the Vietnamese people – to earn the populace's support for the South Vietnam government and turn them against the Viet Cong. Although we were a Navy team, we had little-to-nothing to do with the Navy. We lived with a U.S. Army Special Forces unit. They provided our security but, for our mission, we were accountable to the U.S. Agency for International Development. It was an odd arrangement.

The medical conditions we saw in Vietnam were unorthodox by western standards. Almost daily, our team performed surgical amputations resulting from war trauma. Tuberculosis was endemic and many patients we saw had massive intestinal parasites. We frequently had patients in the hospital with tetanus, and we had a brief outbreak of plague. My experiences in Vietnam, caring for a civilian population in a war zone, prepared me for my work decades later in Afghanistan. Substitute Afghans for Vietnamese and Taliban for Viet Cong and there is a sense of déjà vu.

After completing my tour in Vietnam, I continued my career with the Navy but, until my retirement a few years later, I was only assigned to duty stations and schools in the States. In 1972, the Navy sent me to The Ohio State University, where I got my master's degree in hospital and health system management.

I retired from the Navy in 1978, after twenty-two years of active duty service. My first job out of the Navy was as the chief operating officer at Vanderbilt University Hospital, a 625-bed academic medical center in Nashville, Tennessee. I managed all the day-to-day operations of that complex organization during a time when we were constructing the first phase of a new health sciences campus. Five years later, I was recruited from Vanderbilt to be the chief operating officer of Baystate Medical Center in Springfield, Massachusetts. Baystate was a three-hospital academic center. It was the second largest hospital in New England and was the western campus of Tufts University School of Medicine. When we acquired a fourth hospital on the Vermont border, I became CEO of the three-hospital complex in Springfield and executive vice president of the four-hospital system. The positions at Vanderbilt and Baystate enabled me to acquire new skills beyond those I developed in the Navy, and I gained experience managing large and complex academic medical centers.

I realized I was privileged to have held such prominent positions in the American health care system, but in just a few short years I knew it wasn't how I wanted to spend my life and career. It was no surprise that the majority of my time was spent dealing with finances – budgets and bottom-lines. I felt out of touch with the people I thought we existed to serve. I increasingly knew my heart wasn't in my jobs and I began to consider other options.

In 1987, I accepted an offer from the executive search firm Heidrick & Struggles to join them in their Boston office as a *headhunter*, an executive search consultant. I worked in that position for nearly five years, conducting searches for hospital chief executives, and university deans and presidents. I became co-managing partner of the company's health care practice and quickly moved from the entry role of consultant to partner. I was eventually selected to be a director of the company. There were both rewarding and frustrating aspects of the job but, once again, the job wasn't giving me the personal and professional satisfaction I wanted – and I still yearned to travel and work abroad. A pattern was developing that didn't look very promising. I wasn't sure where life was taking me.

In early 1991, one of my colleagues in our Boston office was contacted by representatives of the Aga Khan University, in Karachi

Pakistan, and invited to participate in a *shootout* to conduct a search for someone to fill the position of director general and chief executive officer of the University's 650-bed hospital. A shootout is macho headhunter jargon for a competitive presentation against other search firms. My colleague had previously placed an American in the position of Dean and Acting Rector at the University, so he was a good prospect to do a search for the hospital CEO. He asked me if I would like to go on the shootout with him.

Did I? Of course I did. The international element of the search was appealing to me. I asked, "If we're selected to do the search won't one of us have to go to Karachi to get started on it?"

"Absolutely Lee – and if we do get the search you should be the one to go. I had a terrible experience when I was there before. I lost the heel off my shoe, I broke the zipper on my fly, and I got diarrhea. I don't give a damn if I ever go to Karachi again."

In preparation for the shootout, I reviewed material about AKU and Karachi that had been collected during the earlier search. I think my decisive moment came while Pat and I were at our home in Massachusetts watching a video of an AKU graduation ceremony. I watched with fascination as a Mercedes-Benz carrying then Prime Minister of Pakistan Benazir Bhutto, the ceremony's chief guest speaker, pulled up at the end of a red carpet leading to the entrance of a *shamiana* – an enormous tent – where the event would be held. The students and faculty were resplendent in their convocation garb. The exotic music and elegance of the event and setting swept me away.

"I want that job," I proclaimed.

Pat's response was astute. "I wondered how long it would take for you to say that," she said.

I had several offers to leave consulting and return to running hospitals during my years as a consultant with Heidrick & Struggles, but none of them appealed to me. I felt I would just be returning to what I had previously found to be unfulfilling. This was different. This was in Karachi, Pakistan.

I asked my partner what he thought about me applying for the position. He was surprised at my interest in it. "There's no doubt you are professionally qualified for the job, Lee. You're more than qualified for it. I don't think that's the issue you have to consider. This job will not be like anything you've ever done before. That place is a world apart from your life here."

Without realizing it, he had just sealed the deal in my mind. Now I was even more certain I wanted the job.

We agreed that we would make a genuine pitch for Heidrick & Struggles to do the search, but then I would privately express my personal interest in the position. When I was alone with the University team, I said I would like them to consider me for the position and, if they did, Heidrick & Struggles would take itself out of consideration to do the search. I gave them my résumé and suggested they could either hire me outright or, if they wished, they could select another search firm and put me on the slate to be compared with other candidates. They were taken aback at the turn of events. A headhunter didn't fit their ideal criteria for someone to be their hospital's CEO.

After reviewing my résumé they called me the next morning and said they would like to meet with me. After a couple of hours' discussion they said they wouldn't select me outright but they would like me to be a candidate. They chose another firm that conducted an international search. In the end they hired me. My long-standing desire to return to work in the international arena was about to come true.

While it was my wish to live and work abroad, it was not quite the same for Pat. Before I offered myself as a candidate we had many thoughtful – I should say *heavy* – discussions about what it would mean in our lives. Despite my naval career and my own travels abroad in the Navy, moving to Karachi would be our first occasion to live together outside the United States. There were overseas Navy postings where Pat would have enjoyed living abroad with me – maybe someplace sunny and nice like Italy or Spain, or even a place as different as Japan – but Karachi? It was testimony to her love and support for me, and her understanding of my passion for the experience, that she agreed to it. Leaving our family behind and moving to a place as distant and different as Karachi took great courage on her part.

KARACHI AND THE AKDN

Pat and I arrived in Karachi for the first time in January 1992, a few months after the first Gulf War in Iraq, known as *Operation Desert Storm*. There was some anti-American sentiment in Pakistan during that war, but not too much. Generally, relations were pretty good between the U.S. and Pakistan in those days and Pakistanis were friendly toward Americans.

In the early nineties, most international flights arrived in Karachi early in the morning. Our first impression of Karachi was its distinctive smell. It enveloped us as soon as we walked out of the airport terminal. In one powerful package it conveyed the sour odor of sweat on countless unwashed human bodies; the pungent stink of ripe garbage; and the distant scent of unidentified large animals. I'm sure many visitors would find it offensive. Strangely, I didn't. Maybe my early life working amidst strong smells on a farm made it more familiar to me.

By the time we arrived at our hotel it was about 4.30 a.m. After briefly settling in we walked onto the balcony outside our tenth-floor room. The pre-dawn darkness was illuminated by endless constellations and strings of amber lights crisscrossing and merging into one another through neighborhoods and on distant horizons. Daily activities hadn't yet begun and the city was silent. Suddenly the stillness was broken by the amplified sounds of

muezzins, men who call Muslims to prayer, simultaneously calling the faithful to their morning prayer all across the city. From
every direction we heard the musical Arabic chant of the Adhan:

> *Allahu Akbar (God is Greatest)*
> I witness that there is no god but Allah
> I witness that Muhammad is the Messenger of God
> Rise up for prayer
> Rise up for salvation
> Prayer is better than sleep
> God is greatest
> There is no god but God.

To Muslims the sound of prayer calls reverberating across the landscape must be as familiar and comforting as the sound of church
bells ringing is to Christian ears, even more so because they hear
it five times every day. Like church bells, the muezzin's melodic
chant resonates and hangs in the air long after each phrase is ut-
tered. We had just arrived in Karachi from the Christmas season
in Yankee Boston. This was definitely not a church-bell world. If
we wanted to experience something different, this was going to
be it.

Karachi is Pakistan's largest city by a wide margin. There are so
many people living in its *katchi abadis*, unsanctioned shanty-
towns, that it is doubtful anybody really knows its true population. In the mid-1990s, estimates ranged from twelve to fifteen
million. More recent estimates are as high as twenty million. Few
would doubt that it is one of the world's *megacities*.

Our lives were quickly filled with adventure and discovery. Pat
became absorbed in the intensity of daily life and I became

immersed in my work. We formed close and supportive relationships with expatriates and Pakistanis. We traveled freely around the country and we were comfortable shopping in markets and wandering through chaotic bazaars, haggling over prices of everything from household necessities to oriental carpets and brass.

Working at AKU was a rewarding experience for me. It is one of the extraordinary institutions of the developing world. No one who visits there leaves unimpressed. It was founded in 1983 by His Highness Prince Karim Aga Khan IV, the 49th and current Imam of the Shia Imami Nizari Ismaili Muslims. According to some estimates, Ismailis number about fifteen to twenty million worldwide. They constitute the second largest Shia community in the Muslim world and are scattered in more than twenty-five countries and on multiple continents including Asia, Africa, Europe, and North America. More than a thousand years ago, in 970 AD, one of His Highness' ancestors founded Al-Azhar University in Cairo, the oldest continuously operating university in the world.

While His Highness is foremost a spiritual leader of Ismailis, he is also a humanitarian, a philanthropist, and a corporate executive. He bridges cultures of the East and West. He has created, and oversees, an international network of institutions involved in fields ranging from education, health, and rural development, to architecture and the promotion of private sector enterprise. There is nothing starry-eyed or utopian about his view of how to bring about constructive change in unstable societies. His institutions' practices and programs are founded in the gritty realism of functional and transparent political structures, integrity in governance, and inclusiveness.

When I accepted the roles of director general and CEO of the University hospital, I also accepted the responsibility to lead it in pursuit of the goal to be the premier teaching hospital in Pakistan. I arrived just before its tenth anniversary. In those early days, the hospital was struggling to achieve the level of performance originally envisioned for it. Its inpatient bed capacity was 654 but, in 1992, only about 350 beds were opened. While it was the principal teaching site for a school of medicine and a school of nursing, it only offered secondary level care and no tertiary, or subspecialty care, in any of its services. We implemented the first genuinely tertiary service: open-heart surgery in 1993. By 1998, we had implemented multiple advanced care services and subspecialty training programs, and the hospital was undisputedly recognized as the premier teaching hospital in Pakistan.

Working at the AKU finally gave me the personal rewards and satisfaction I had not found in any of my jobs since leaving the Navy. I was able to apply skills I had learned at academic centers in the United States in delivering care to a population that had no other local opportunities for care of an international standard. The staff I worked with was as dedicated and eager to learn as any I had ever known, and the results of our improvements in care were more immediately apparent than they were in hospitals I worked at in the States.

While Pat and I had interesting and rewarding lives, living and working in Karachi was challenging. The place is a cauldron of political and ethnic conflict. Karachi and Sindh, its province, are homes to a large population of *Mohajirs* – literally, people who came from someplace else. Mohajirs are Urdu-speaking Muslims who migrated to Pakistan from India in 1947. In Punjab and the Northwest Frontier Province, migrant Urdu-speaking populations were absorbed into the local cultures but, in Sindh, assimilation did not take place, particularly in the urban areas. The indigenous Sindh population was mostly rural, so in major cities the Mohajirs assumed a dominant status. This led to cultural and political tensions between ethnic Sindhis and the Mohajirs. The Mohajirs formed their own political party in 1984 – the *Mohajir Qaumi Movement* (MQM), which became a competitive political force in urban Sindh, in opposition to the Bhutto-led Pakistan Peoples' Party. That was a recipe for trouble.

We had only been in Karachi for six months when the Pakistan Army launched *Operation Clean-Up*. The declared goal of the operation was to cleanse the city of *anti-social elements*, but the main target was the MQM. The justification for the operation was the so-called *Jinnahpur Affair*, an alleged plot by Urdu-speaking Mohajirs to make Karachi an autonomous state and their homeland. It was a time of intense violence in the city involving urban guerrilla warfare between the MQM and the Army. It is regarded as one of the bloodiest periods in Karachi's history.

By the mid-nineties, Karachi morning newspapers frequently reported twenty-five to thirty murders the previous night. The MQM declared strike days almost weekly – days on which they shut down the city's businesses and transportation. Motorcyclists would ride through the streets firing Kalashnikovs into the air and into store fronts to warn residents and business owners to observe the strike and stay inside. There were thirty-three strike days in Karachi in 1995. Two of our University buses were hijacked while transporting employees. The employees were ordered off the buses and, in one instance, the driver was beaten and the bus burned. The hospital always remained open and in full operation despite the threats and risks of danger. Many of the staff would walk more than five miles, disregarding their personal safety, to get to work. Some were Ismailis, and their dedication was partly fueled by loyalty to their Imam's institution. For all of them, it was due to their professionalism and dedication to ensure continuity of care for patients they knew depended on them. I greatly admired their selflessness and tried every way I could to let them know how much I appreciated their courageous commitment to the hospital.

Karachi is known for its late night social activity but, during this time, people would return to their homes by early evening. It wasn't safe to stay on the streets. Surprisingly, morale within the expatriate community remained high. The way they faced this kind of adversity reminded me of the way members of military communities living overseas supported one another. Pat and I were privileged to have support systems both within the expatriate and Pakistani communities.

It wasn't as if we were isolated and held captive in Karachi. We could get away when we felt it necessary. Regions of Pakistan outside Karachi were stable and peaceful in those days. We could drive into the interior of Sindh Province, and we could easily get on a plane and fly to other fascinating cities like Lahore and Peshawar. We could visit places with breathtaking scenery like the Khyber Pass, the Swat Valley, and the Himalayan foothills. Other get-away opportunities came within the AKDN itself. The University's board of trustees frequently met with His Highness in France. I attended those meetings at least two or three times per year to represent the hospital's affairs. Pat always accompanied me. We explored and came to love Paris and the French countryside, and at least a couple of times each year, the AKDN health sector held meetings in India and East Africa. We relished the opportunities to travel to those locations. It was almost an overdose of diverse and exotic cultures.

A sizeable community of Americans lived and worked in Karachi during most of the time we were there – at AKU, at the international Karachi American School, in oil industry companies, and at the U.S. Consulate. Those people were all experienced at living abroad. We socialized together and had strong bonds. Despite the nightly violence, Pat and her expatriate friends were comfortable going on daytime outings into back street areas of the city, shopping for local artifacts.

Then things began to change. During the peak of violence in 1995, two American U.S. Consulate employees, neighbors of ours, were attacked and murdered on their way to work, and a third was wounded. The perpetrators of that attack, and the reasons for it, were never known. Whoever was behind it, that tragedy shocked the entire expatriate community and caused Americans to take cover. Suddenly we weren't as willing to roam the city as we were before. Four more Americans were assassinated in 1997 – employees of Union Texas Petroleum, a Houston-based oil company operating in Pakistan. Like the earlier Consulate employees, they were attacked on their way to work in a scenario almost identical to the one in 1995. The drama of both of these experiences was intense for me. In both instances, the bodies of the dead Americans were brought to the University Hospital to be kept in our morgue until arrangements could be made for their transportation back to the States. Pat and I found ourselves in the midst of a grieving and anxious American community, of which many members were our close friends.

The U.S. Consulate drastically reduced its presence in Karachi after the second assassination event and relocated most of its services and staff to Islamabad. Union Texas moved its corporate staff out of Pakistan to Dubai, in the United Arab Emirates. Their departure strongly affected Pat and me. It's remarkable how fast a social climate can turn around from one that is warm and welcoming to one that is cold and empty. Suddenly we felt very alone. We had stayed in Karachi longer than we intended when I first took the job, and I had more than fulfilled my commitments. We decided it was time for us to move on, as well.

I wasn't sure what I would do next. I was approaching sixty. I intended to keep working, but other than a desire to remain involved in the international healthcare field I didn't have any definite objectives. I began looking for opportunities, primarily in Southeast Asia. When His Highness learned that I was planning to leave, he invited me to join his Secretariat staff in France. He wanted me to oversee the Network's entire hospital system, including hospitals in East Africa, Pakistan, and India. I jumped on it. The opportunity to live in France and be involved with the Network's hospitals in Africa and Asia was too good to pass up.

Pat and I moved to Paris in 1998 and I began work at His Highness' estate, called *Aiglemont* (Eagle Mountain), located near the charming village of Chantilly, about thirty miles north of Paris. At Aiglemont I was exposed to the AKDN's much broader social sector and economic development agenda including schools, housing, tourism, media, insurance, and banking. I saw the Network from both its philanthropic and entrepreneurial sides. Its scope and breadth are unparalleled among the world's private development organizations.

My duties involved overseeing the activities of hospitals owned and managed by Aga Khan Health Services, one of the AKDN's social welfare enterprises. Aga Khan Health Services is one of the most comprehensive private not-for-profit health care systems in the developing world. It operates 325 health facilities, including nine hospitals, in Central and South Asia, as well as East Africa. I served on the governing bodies of Aga Khan hospitals and health systems in Kenya, Tanzania, and Uganda. I worked closely with the Prince Aly Khan Hospital in Bombay (now Mumbai), India, and I continued my involvement with the University Hospital in Karachi. We had construction projects underway at our hospitals in Nairobi, Kenya, and Dar es Salaam, Tanzania during this period, and we were planning future hospitals in Northern Pakistan and Central Asia. If I could have written the script for my life this would have been it, but I would have thought it too much to expect.

I never worked in Afghanistan during my years at either Karachi or Aiglemont, but I did some work in Tajikistan, another country bordering Afghanistan. Shortly after I arrived in France, I was asked to go to Tajikistan and develop a plan for improvement of health services in Khorog, the capital city of Gorno-Badakhshan *oblast*, or province. Khorog sits in the Pamir mountain range, just across Afghanistan's northern border. It is an area of interest to the AKDN because a large population of Ismailis, followers of the Aga Khan, lives there.

When the Soviet Union dissolved in 1991, its former Republics suddenly had new-found independence. This wasn't a good deal for all of them. Tajikistan, for example, fell into civil war and experienced fighting and political instability throughout the mid-nineties. The effect on its civil society was severe and its economy was devastated. Tens of thousands of Tajiks were killed and more than half a million were displaced. A peace agreement was finally brokered in 1997 and, for the first time since Tajikistan's independence, some order was restored.

One of the Tajikistan populations most affected during the civil war was the *Pamir* – the people of Gorno-Badakhshan, many of whom were Ismailis. They suffered some of the worst fighting between the government and opposition forces. Several thousand Pamiris are believed to have died. The government attempted a blockage of food, energy, and medical supplies to the region. The Pamiris maintain they would have starved had the AKDN humanitarian aid organization, FOCUS, not provided food to them.

The situation had improved and was stable by the time I visited Khorog, but the population was still suffering from severe poverty. It was even difficult for them to get crops from the fields to the market because there was no fuel for transport vehicles.

I spent several days in Khorog developing a plan for a state-of-the-art diagnostic and treatment center in the existing, decrepit, Soviet-era public hospital. It would be more than a decade before a version of that plan would be implemented. I didn't know it at the time but my work in Khorog would be relevant to my future work in Afghanistan and, a decade later, I would be back in Tajikistan, still involved in planning its hospital services.

I remained at Aiglemont until mid-2000. By then, Pat and I had lived outside the U.S. for more than eight years. Our lives had been exciting and fulfilling. We had traveled to places we would never have dreamed possible. We had walked in the shadows of the tallest mountains on the planet, we had watched elephants and other big game graze and play in East Africa's Maasai Mara and Serengeti, and we had lived in Paris. We developed friendships that would last the rest of our lives. We were privileged to have had such fascinating opportunities but we had been apart from our family long enough. Matters back in the States required more attention than we could give them from abroad. We decided it was time to return home. When I left the Network I didn't know that in just a few short years the AKDN, Afghanistan, Pakistan, Tajikistan, and East Africa would all once again play important roles in my life.

When I returned to the States, I continued working with an AKDN task force, developing strategies to create an integrated health care system in East Africa. For more than a year, I worked part-time from my new home in Chattanooga, Tennessee. That work ended in late 2001. For the first time in nearly forty-five years, I was not employed full-time and, more importantly, I was not doing work that I felt passionate about. That's what made the call asking, "Lee, how would you like to go to Afghanistan?" all the more welcome.

FIRST VISIT TO
AFGHANISTAN

I arrived in Kabul on July 4, 2004, a few weeks after I got the call from Aiglemont and two-and-a half years after Western allied military forces, led by the U.S., had ousted the Taliban. My arrival had a confused beginning.

Arrangements were made for me to be picked up at the airport by someone on the staff of the Aga Khan Health Services office in Kabul. They were to take me to the Inter-Continental Hotel where I would stay. I walked out of the airport terminal looking for an Asian, probably a Pakistani, who would give some indication he was there to pick me up. Instead, I saw two tall Caucasians holding a sign that read *Hilling*. They were dressed in dark blue fatigue-style uniforms with their trousers bloused in spit-shined black boots. They both wore bullet-proof vests and very large handguns rested in holsters hanging at their sides. This was not the greeting party I had expected.

As I tentatively approached the two imposing figures I heard a voice behind me urgently calling, "Mr. Hilling, Mr. Hilling."

I turned and saw the Pakistani I had expected, running across the parking lot toward us. He was waving a sign that also said *Hilling*.

There ensued a confused discussion. My AKDN colleague was insistent I come with him. The two armed guys – it turned out they were French and spoke no English – were equally insistent I come with them. I could only understand a little of what they were saying, but their non-verbal language was very clear. My choice seemed obvious – go with the guys with guns.

I explained to my AKDN colleague that I would go with the French escorts and work things out later when I knew what was going on. He was not comfortable with that but he reluctantly agreed. To be honest I wasn't comfortable with it either. This was Afghanistan. I was being led away by guys with guns, and I wasn't sure where I would be taken. I hoped I was making the right decision.

My French attendants promptly escorted me across the tarmac to their vehicle: a black, armored Toyota Land Cruiser with darkened windows. Perched on the front of the vehicle's hood was a large communications antenna that reminded me of a rhinoceros horn. I later learned that after Humvees, the mode of transportation used by the allied military forces, this type of vehicle was next in the pecking order on Kabul's streets and roads. It was used to carry high-ranking diplomats and assorted other VIPs and bigwigs, mostly foreigners, to important meetings and places.

Off we went to . . . well, I didn't know where. We assertively maneuvered our way through the chaotic traffic. After a short distance we turned off the street toward a heavily guarded and secured metal gate. It was promptly opened and we were waved through without delay, as if we were important and they were expecting us. We entered a large courtyard. The place was tranquil and quiet, protected from the noise and hubbub of the streets outside. We pulled up in front of a building where a man and a woman stood, apparently awaiting our arrival.

"Bonjour Monsieur Hilling," said the man, then in English, "Welcome to the French Embassy."

The French Embassy! So that's where I was. "Bonjour," I replied.

The man introduced himself as the Cultural Attaché at the Embassy. The woman was the Ambassador's secretary.

They inquired how my trip and been and told me His Highness had contacted the Ambassador and asked him to do whatever he could to assist me while I was in Kabul. The Ambassador, who was not at the Embassy at the moment, assumed I would stay there as his guest.

That was all very lovely, but I did not want to stay at the French Embassy. The restrictions on my movement and demands on my time would probably complicate my freedom to come and go as required for me to accomplish the purposes of my visit.

"Let us show you to your room," my hosts said. Without objecting for the moment, I followed them up the stairs to the second floor of the Ambassador's residence. They led me into a spacious, well-furnished room. A king size bed was fashionably decorated with floral designed spreads and pillows. A basket filled with fresh fruit and chocolates sat on a table beside the bed and a large, ornate antique armoire stood against the wall at the foot of the bed. I could have been at La Meridian Hotel in Paris. I didn't know how my accommodations would be at the Inter-Continental Hotel, but I doubted they could beat this.

I thought I'd better get control of the situation before it went any further. I politely expressed my sincere gratitude for the hospitality, but I explained that other arrangements had been made for my lodging and logistical support during my visit, and I felt I should avail myself of them. Reluctantly they relented and said they would convey my message to the Ambassador. Relieved, I called Aga Khan Health Services and asked them to send transportation to pick me up and take me to the Inter-Continental. My previously rebuffed Pakistani escort arrived within the hour and off we went across town.

Kabul sits just south of the Hindu Kush mountain range. While it is in a valley, its elevation is high, about 5,900 feet. As we wound our way between hills and through traffic I learned what a colorless place Kabul is. There is little greenery and the few trees that do exist are muted in color by coats of brownish gray dust. The city's most striking visual feature is its ubiquitous hillside houses. Starting at street level and ascending upward, every hill or mountain is densely populated with ramshackle mud and stucco houses. They are generally colorless – every now and then a bright pink or blue one boldly stands out – and look like they were carved out of the rocky hillside rather than constructed on it. Only at the highest elevations do dwellings finally dwindle in number and come to an end.

On the surface, Afghanistan seemed stable and peaceful in 2004. We certainly weren't paying much attention to it in the United States. Military operations in Afghanistan were low-level because the U.S. had shifted its attention to Iraq, where it launched a complex and all-consuming war. The *war*, as it was, in Afghanistan consisted of the allied forces conducting military operations to eradicate, or at least contain, a resurging Taliban. They were also purportedly still trying to track down Osama bin Laden.

Afghanistan was far from secure in 2004. There were frequent military troop casualties, albeit not in the numbers being incurred in Iraq. Civilians -- both Afghans and foreign humanitarian aid workers -- were also being killed. In June, the Taliban killed five workers of *Médecins Sans Frontières, Doctors Without Borders*, in the north-western province of Badghis. Médecins Sans Frontières is one of the most heroic and humanitarian organizations in the world. Its credo is "We find out where conditions are the worst – the places others are *not* going – and that's where we want to be." That fearless organization was in the process of withdrawing from Afghanistan at the very time I arrived in Kabul. By August, all of its medical projects there were closed. It had worked in the country for almost twenty-four years. It was unsettling to me that, just as I was arriving, such a courageous organization was in the process of leaving.

Afghanistan was at war for decades. In 1979 it was invaded by the Soviet Union. For much of the next decade, the U.S., Pakistan, and Saudi-backed Mujahidin forces fought the Soviets in one of the pivotal events leading to the end of the Cold War. When the Soviets were eventually defeated and withdrew their combat forces from Afghanistan in 1989, they left behind a puppet regime, the Marxist People's Democratic Party of Afghanistan, headed by Mohammad Najibullah Ahmadzai, simply referred to as Najibullah.

The rival Mujahidin factions remained somewhat united until they toppled the Najibullah regime in April 1992 – just about the time Pat and I were settling into Karachi, next door in Pakistan. After they eliminated their common enemy, the factions then turned on one another. For the next four years warlords and their militias, characterized by religion, ethnicity, and region – Gulbuddin

Hekmatyar's radical Islamists, Abdul Rashid Dostum's Uzbeks, Ahmed Shah Massoud's Tajiks, Abdul Ali Mazari's Hazaras – and others – engaged in a free-for-all for dominance.

By the mid-nineties the Mujahidin had beaten themselves sense-less. They fought one another, terrorized Afghanistan's populace, and destroyed the economy and infrastructure of the country – yet none was able to gain dominance, and none was willing to com-promise with its rivals. This era of atrocities led many Afghans to initially welcome the relative "peace" that came with the Taliban. From the early- to mid-1990s, the warring Mujahidin forces killed thousands of civilians in Kabul and devastated most of the city. The United Nations estimated that ninety percent of Kabul's buildings were damaged or destroyed.

Kabul was under nearly total military occupation in 2004. I was struck by the city's Spartan ugliness and disorder resulting from the preoccupation with security. Endless coils of barbed-wire were strung atop walls, protecting military installations, govern-mental ministries, hotels, and posh new residences from would-be invaders.

Our drive through the city was slow. Geography and security conspired to create vehicular gridlock. Traffic circumnavigating the city's many hills inevitably converged at bottle-neck points. Frequent barricades and restricted traffic patterns imposed by the military caused illogical and disruptive circulation patterns, winding through and around maze-like concrete barriers, always under the suspicious glares of police or security forces. Noisy, fume-spewing vehicles crisscrossed in each other's paths, their drivers blowing horns and jockeying for position. The Aga Khan Health Services vehicle was neither as imposing nor as assertive as the one that transported me to the French Embassy. I could only watch as the vehicles with rhino horn antennas, police vehicles, and military vehicles all bullied their way through traffic with self-assumed authority.

Despite the bedlam, I sensed a modicum of traffic etiquette. Women covered from head to toe in flowing pale blue burkahs (often guided by a child), vendors pushing or pulling their carts, and beggars were all granted slight leeway in wending their way through the swarm of vehicles. More able-bodied and agile pedestrians were left to bob and weave through the gauntlet of traffic at their own risk.

Stark evidence of war and destruction was everywhere. Hulks of burned and twisted vehicles sat on vacant lots. Buildings were scarred from assault by mortars, rockets, and gunfire. Skeletal walls stood like sentries beside piles of rubble that were floors and ceilings in another time. We passed a former cinema – a large sign saying *Cinema* was still intact on its front. In its heyday it was probably one of Kabul's main entertainment venues. Now it had no roof. Between heavily damaged exterior walls I could see a staircase spiraling upward. It must have once led patrons to a balcony from which they watched Bollywood movies. Now it led to nowhere, like a scene lifted from a Dali painting.

We passed a school for boys, where classes were in session. The front wall was completely missing and all the interior contents and occupants were visible to passersby. I could see boys climbing up and down the steps and sitting at their desks. I thought if they weren't careful they would lose their balance and fall to the ground below. The place reminded me of a dollhouse with one of its sides exposed to enable little hands to reach in and play with dolls and furniture. In this structure the occupants were animated and moved themselves.

Across the street from the school was a completely intact three-story business center, seemingly unmarred by the war. A sign atop the building boldly identified it as *The World Trade Center*. That specious taunt caused me to wince.

Mixed with the scenes of devastation were signs of reconstruction and new development. Ostentatious, over-the-top houses were being constructed by the new Kabul wealthy – warlords, drug lords, and Afghans clever enough to tap into the massive amount of international military and aid money flowing into the economy. The most flamboyant new emporiums were marriage houses. Multi-storied and flaunting Las Vegas-style flashy neon adornments, those palaces of connubial rites were rapidly becoming the foremost additions to the cityscape.

We finally arrived at the Inter-Continental Hotel, perched on a hill near the western edge of the city. We followed the road up the hill, passing a couple of casually-guarded security checkpoints. There were no luxury hotels in Kabul in 2004. Most accommodations were in guesthouses, mainly private residences transformed to accommodate visitors. The Inter-Continental was the closest thing to luxury lodging the city had to offer at the time. It suffered extensive damage and fell into disrepair during the civil war. By the time I arrived it had been extensively renovated and returned to international standards – well, sort of. At the entrance to the lobby was a sign declaring NO WEAPONS in both Dari and English. That was reassuring.

THE FRENCH HOSPITAL

The next morning, I got an early start on my work. I had a lot to accomplish in a short amount of time. The first thing I wanted to do was physically assess the hospital being built by La Chaîne. I needed to know as much as possible about it, including how it would serve the needs of Afghans and how Afghan government officials felt about it. I also wanted to know what they thought about the AKDN's potential involvement with it.

I knew from my advance research that, after decades of war, Afghanistan's health system and the health status of its people were in a terrible state. A 2002 United Nations Human Development report ranked Afghanistan second-to-last in the world. A World Health Organization study the same year found that Afghanistan's maternal and child health status was among the worst in the world and, in some cases, was the worst. Its child mortality rate was the fourth highest in the world: one in four children died before reaching the age of five. Its maternal mortality rate was the second highest in the world: one in fifteen women died in childbirth. A 2004 article published in the British medical journal *Lancet* reported that Badakhshan Province, in the northeast of the country, had 6,500 maternal deaths per 100,000 births. This was the worst rate ever reported. Dr. Ferozudeen Feroz, Afghanistan's Deputy Minister of Public Health, was blunt in his assessment,

"Afghanistan today has the worst health indicators in the world. We have a horrible situation – a surrealistic situation. Much of today's dilemma is the result of years of war and devastation, both natural and man-made. Now we have to respond to these dire needs for health care."

These conditions did not bode well for the health of women and children in Afghanistan. On the other hand, it seemed a good case could be made for a high quality hospital dedicated to the care of mothers and children.

The hospital was being built in a sector of Kabul called Aliabad, not far from the Inter-Continental Hotel. It hardly seemed possible but the scenes of destruction in Aliabad were worse than anything I had seen while riding through town the previous day. All the warring Mujahidin factions contributed to Kabul's destruction, but one of the worst was the Hezb-e-Islami leader, Gulbuddin Hekmatyar. He was relentless in his attacks and he deliberately targeted civilian areas. Aliabad and the southwestern sector of the city had especially suffered from his attacks. The area's primary inhabitants were Hazaras, mainly Shiite Muslims. They were a frequent target of Sunni and ethnic Pashtu factions in Kabul and elsewhere during the civil war.

Before I sought out anybody at the construction site, I surveyed the sights around it. Kabul Medical University's main administrative building was located just to the south. The building's walls and what once must have been the University's most prominent feature, an ornate bell tower, were pitted and cratered by bullets and mortar shells. To the north, behind the construction site, one of Kabul's hillside communities sprawled upward. The houses were crammed together and appeared to be built on top of one another. I later learned this hill was a vantage point from which Hekmatyar and other militants lobbed rockets down on the University and community below. Immediately to the west was the once esteemed Aliabad Surgical Hospital, or what remained of it. Built seventy years earlier, it was Afghanistan's oldest teaching hospital. Chunks of the building's exterior walls were blown away. Two wings, each three stories high, extended from a once stately but now badly damaged rotunda. Squatters' ragged and dirty sheets and linens hung over balcony railings. It was a sorry state for a former institution of national pride.

So this was FMIC's neighborhood. I felt saddened by so much evidence of violence, hate, and destruction. I wondered if any good could come from it.

The hospital's contractor was *Bouygues*, one of France's leading construction companies. I found Bouygues' onsite managers. They led me on a tour of the site and showed me facility drawings. The drawings were in French. The construction managers and I barely spoke one another's languages, but with effort we successfully struggled through my orientation. They informed me that the ultimate plan was to build a 154-bed Women and Children's Hospital. The facility being built was already referred to in Kabul as the *Mother and Child Hospital* and in France as *Hôpital Meres et Enfants*. The project would be done in two phases. The phase under construction now was designed to be a fifty-eight bed hospital dedicated to pediatric care, primarily pediatric surgery. A second phase, a high-risk maternity center, was planned but not yet funded. The building's dimensions and layout appeared more than adequate to house the intended programs. I especially liked its location proximate to Kabul Medical University. That would hopefully enable collaboration between the institutions.

Later in the day, I finally met the French Ambassador. He invited me to the Embassy for a private lunch. We dined in a spacious room, the centerpiece of which was an impressive grand piano. Floor-to-ceiling sliding glass doors led from our dining area to a patio and garden outside. Bastille Day was just a few days away and groundskeepers were sprucing up the grounds for special ceremonies that would be held at the Embassy. Our meal was classic French cuisine accompanied by a delicious wine. In light of such elegance and hospitality I reconsidered whether I should have accepted the earlier offer to stay there. Oh well, too late now.

The Ambassador told me the hospital project had very high visibility in France, but he was concerned about the way it was proceeding. "La Chaîne has raised money for it from the public-at-large in France and they have attracted prominent celebrities and political and civic leaders' support for it," he said. "If it doesn't go well, I'm concerned this Embassy will be left holding the bag."

His comments concerned me. "Does that mean you don't support it?" I asked. "Without your support I'm concerned about the AKDN getting involved with it."

"Mais non," he said. "You can be assured the French government and my Embassy is committed to provide funds for training Afghan doctors in France and for training by French doctors visiting Kabul. My concern is that La Chaîne will not be able to manage it. I'm glad the AKDN might become involved. I know of their experience and expertise in managing programs in Afghanistan and elsewhere in the developing world and I would be very comfortable if they were partners in the project."

Those remarks certainly gave me something to think about. If the

AKDN was to become involved, the commitment of the French government was crucial. His high regard for the Network was reassuring.

Over the next few days I met with high-ranking Afghan government officials. They expressed strong support for the hospital and AKDN's involvement with it. Some went further and expressed their desire for the AKDN to take a leadership role in developing and improving management of other Ministry of Public Health hospitals in Kabul. The Deputy Minister of Public Health, complained, "There is not one well-managed hospital in Kabul."

The Dean of Kabul Medical University was concerned about the lack of teaching hospitals. "Before the war," he said, "Kabul Medical University had five teaching hospitals, now we have none and our graduates are unable to get clinical experience. We have 3,200 students and 200 faculty but we have no teaching hospitals. It is good that the French hospital will focus on care for mothers and children, but we need more than that. We need access to a larger and more complex hospital for teaching." He welcomed the Aga Khan University's involvement in Afghanistan, "AKU is famous and has lots of friends in Afghanistan."

If the AKDN decided to become involved with the French hospital, it wouldn't be the Network's first venture into Afghanistan. It was already heavily invested in the country. The Aga Khan Fund for Economic Development, a company within the AKDN, had two very visible projects. It launched Roshan, a telecommunications company in 2003. Roshan quickly became Afghanistan's leading telecommunications operator, covering over sixty percent of the population and connecting five million active subscribers in 230 cities and towns across the country's thirty-four provinces.

Within just a few years, Roshan was reportedly Afghanistan's largest private investor, and its tax payments contributed approximately five percent of the Afghan government's revenue.

Another prominent AKDN project launched in 2004 was the Kabul Serena Hotel. That ambitious undertaking entailed restoring and expanding the Kabul Hotel, a former center-city landmark originally built in 1945. A burgeoning international community of diplomatic, development, and aid organizations were frequently visiting Kabul, but there was a dearth of hotel accommodations. President Karzai approached His Highness to help restore Kabul's hotel capacity so that visitors traveling to Kabul would have acceptable accommodation. The Kabul Serena was an addition to an already prestigious international chain of Serena Hotels in Africa and South and Central Asia.

The AKDN was also involved in Afghanistan's social sector. Aga Khan Health Services, operating under a public-private partnership agreement with the Government of Afghanistan, already managed the Bamyan Provincial Hospital and the primary care health systems in Bamyan, Badakhshan, and Baghlan Provinces. If the AKDN decided to accept the invitation to be involved with this project, I assumed Aga Khan Health Services would be the entity eventually assigned responsibility to represent it in the partnership. I later learned that assumption was wrong.

Shortly before wrapping up my visit in Kabul, I received a call from Aiglemont telling me that His Highness would be in Kabul at the same time and he wanted to meet with me. We hadn't seen one another since I left his staff at Aiglemont nearly four years earlier. Arrangements were made for us to meet at the Presidential Palace compound.

I arrived there late in the afternoon. His Highness had been meeting dignitaries and diplomats in a room set aside for him. I was escorted in to meet him. He greeted me warmly and was eager to know my early impressions about the proposed partnership. Not unexpectedly, his questions went right to the crux of the matter, with an eye to the future and on the big picture: Should we seriously consider the opportunity and, if so, under what terms? Was the French vision sound? Would the project serve the needs of Afghans? What about future phases of development? What about the adequacy of land for expansion? What about the ongoing human resources need? What were the economics of the project?

Luckily, I had learned enough in the previous few days to have developed some thoughts on most of those matters. I told him I believed there was strong support for the hospital and AKDN's involvement with it. I said that if the AKDN had any interest in either owning or being involved with a tertiary care hospital in Afghanistan then the opportunity had merit to consider. He informed me that, under the right circumstances, the AKDN vision in Afghanistan conceivably went beyond just providing care in a single hospital. It could involve medical education and research and include AKU. Moreover, a Kabul-based hospital might play a central role in a regional network of hospitals and health facilities that reached out to Afghan provinces and beyond – across the border to Tajikistan.

A surprising and pleasant outcome of our meeting was that he asked if I would consider continuing to work with the Network as a consultant. If so, he would like to call on me for future work on this project. I couldn't have been happier. I said I would definitely like that.

I was scheduled to travel to France after I finished my work in Kabul. I would meet with La Chaîne leadership in Paris and then make a written report to His Highness. It appeared, based on our conversation in Kabul, that this could be just the beginning of a long-term engagement for me. It felt good to be back.

THE FRENCH
CONNECTION

I flew from Kabul to France on July 11, 2004. I first went to Aiglemont and then took the train to Paris to meet with the La Chaîne team. I love Paris. When Pat and I lived there my job required that I travel so much that we didn't have the opportunity to fully enjoy all the city had to offer. Since I left Aiglemont and we moved back to the States we had only returned once to Paris. On that occasion, we rented an apartment for two weeks in the Champs-Élysées district, not far from where we lived when I worked at Aiglemont. In those two weeks we engaged in a veritable feast of Paris' delights. We attended a concert of Vivaldi's Four Seasons at the magnificent La Sainte Chapelle; we saw a performance of Wagner's Flying Dutchman at the Opera Bastille; we went to museums and more museums; we drank pitchers of red wine at sidewalk cafes in the Latin Quarter; we savored rum and raisin ice cream while walking on the Avenue des Champs-Élysées; and we ate in as many of our favorite restaurants as we could manage. What's not to like about Paris!

It was great to be back but my visit this time would be all business. La Chaîne's offices were located on the south side of Paris on the sprawling compound of *Hôpital Broussais*. They weren't close to where I exited the subway and I wasn't exactly sure where I was going. By the time I wound my way through the neighborhood streets and the hospital grounds, I was late for our meeting.

When I arrived I was led to a conference room where a small group of people awaited me. I was introduced first to La Chaîne's president, Professor Alain Deloche. With his silver-gray hair and sonorous voice, his demeanor and personality matched his status as an academic and his distinction as one of France's most prominent heart surgeons. He graciously welcomed me and assured me that my tardy arrival was no problem.

I was introduced to the rest of the La Chaîne team. That was my first occasion to meet Jean-Roch Serra and Dr. Eric Cheysson. Jean-Roch Serra was, at that time, the organization's treasurer. He was a retired businessman, the former chief executive of the medical equipment company Siemens-France. Eric Cheysson was introduced as president of La Chaîne's Kabul-based operating company, *Enfants Afghans*. That was the entity registered in Afghanistan and responsible for operation of the hospital. I learned Eric was also the chief of a sixty-bed cardiovascular surgery service at the *Hôpital René Dubois* in Pontoise, just outside Paris. I was impressed. If La Chaîne was to become AKDN's partner in Kabul it was clearly represented by a distinguished and accomplished group of individuals. I didn't know it at the time, but for the next several years of my life I would spend countless hours working with many of the people I was meeting here, especially Eric and Jean-Roch.

After espresso and cookies were served, Alain told me how pleased they were that the AKDN was willing to consider the possibility of a partnership with La Chaîne. He asked how much I knew about their organization.

"Not much," I said. "I have some material that you shared with the AKDN earlier, but it didn't tell me a lot of what I need to know."

I didn't say that the hospital business plans I had seen, plans that were prepared by La Chaîne, hadn't made much sense to me. I'd get to that at some point, but at the outset I was more interested in exploring the potential cultural fit between La Chaîne and the AKDN than I was in the details of the hospital's possible business case. If we went far enough in exploring the partnership I knew we would eventually end up developing new business plans. I asked them to tell me about their organization.

La Chaîne de l'Espoir translates from French to English as *The Chain of Hope*. Alain and Eric co-founded the organization in 1988. Their intent was to provide care to the poorest children in developing countries. They started by raising money to pay for medical treatment missions to Europe. By 1998, they had flown more than 1,000 children to Europe from countries where the required treatment was not available. Soon, however, they realized that approach wasn't as effective as it could be. They decided their impact could be greater if they treated children and trained local surgeons in their home countries.

With that new vision they began seeking private partners and companies to fund and build hospitals in countries where there was the greatest need. They had already developed two centers: the *Institute of the Heart* in Maputo, Mozambique, and the *Cardiovascular Center of Phnom Penh,* in Kampuchea, Cambodia. Another cardiac surgery center was in the works in Ho Chi Minh City, Vietnam.

La Chaîne de l'Espoir-France is the founding member of *Surgeons of Hope*, an international network of non-profit medical partners based in several countries. They all share the vision of "curing and training to cure", and the goal of "training local staff while also caring for impoverished children who suffer serious but curable pathologies." Their motto is: "It's not what we bring; it's what we leave behind". I found that statement appealing.

La Chaîne's history and the personalities involved with it had their roots in two other organizations, Médecins Sans Frontières and Médecins du Monde. The main links among the organizations were Alain, Eric, and the French political figure and diplomat, Dr. Bernard Kouchner. In 1971, Kouchner and Alain co-founded Médecins Sans Frontières, but they left it in 1980 and co-founded a new organization, Médecins du Monde.

The reason for their departure from Médecins Sans Frontières was the election of a new president, Claude Malhuret. Malhuret sparked an internal debate about the philosophy of the organization. It centered on the issue of whether Médecins Sans Frontières should remain neutral when its representatives entered a country for humanitarian reasons, even though the country's government or leaders may have instigated the very conditions causing a humanitarian disaster. That was Malhuret's position. Alternatively, should it play a more activist role and broadly publicize the suffering they saw? That was Kouchner's position.

The disagreement came to a head in 1979 when, without support of the majority of Médecins Sans Frontières, Kouchner led a splinter group to charter a ship called *L'Île de Lumière* ("The Island of Light") to sail to the South China Sea. That mission would provide medical aid to Vietnamese "boat people," refugees from Communism in their homeland. Kouchner intended to involve the media in the mission and publicize the plight of the refugees. It would be the first alliance of doctors and journalists – the doctors to treat and the journalists to publicize. Malhuret did not support that publicity-focused approach.

Eric said it was at this time that he more or less stumbled into what became a long-standing relationship with two of the most important people in his life, Kouchner and Alain. "I was attending my first Médecins Sans Frontières meeting at the very time Bernard stormed out. I was caught completely off guard. I was still a young physician, just a resident in training. I wasn't sure what to do. I followed Bernard and a few others out of the meeting. We went for coffee. Bernard announced 'We are now a new organization – a *Committee un bateau pour Vietnam*'."

Eric speaks English very well, but when he wants to express himself about something he feels passionate about – which is often – he reverts to French. He turned to Jean-Roch and asked for help to express some of his thoughts. He continued in English. "Bernard looked at me and asked, 'What do you do?' I said 'I am a surgeon.' In fact, I was only a student surgeon and had yet to do my first surgery. Bernard said 'Yes, we need a surgeon.' Just like that. It was decided. I went on *L'Île de Lumière* with Bernard and Alain. Normally I would have gone on to become a private surgeon with a big car and all the uniform of a private surgeon. It was for me a real change in my life."

I came to this meeting with no knowledge about La Chaîne and little knowledge about Médecins du Monde, but I had known about Médecins Sans Frontières for a long time and admired it very much Here were people that had not only been involved with all of them, but were founders of them. I asked what the similarities or differences were between La Chaîne and those organizations.

"There are both mission and cultural differences," Eric said. "Médecins Sans Frontières is a very big organization. It is primarily focused on refugees, with an emphasis on logistics. It is possible for Médecins Sans Frontières to have planes at their disposal. Médecins du Monde deals more with the medical and psychiatric problems that remain in a population after conflict. Neither of them focuses on surgical problems. La Chaîne's emphasis is on surgery, but not only surgery. We also focus on a very high level of medicine."

Eric smiled as he continued. "That's the difference in our missions. There are cultural difference too. If you are someplace and you see three persons, one from each of the three organizations, it is easy to tell them apart. The guy from Médecins Sans Frontières wears clothes with *MSF* printed on the back and he has a walkie-talkie. The guy from Médecins du Monde has long hair and wears earrings. The guy from La Chaîne has a clean shirt and sometimes wears a tie. We're not all cut from the same mold."

That was a pretty graphic description. I asked, "So you see yourselves more as institution builders? I guess that's consistent with the motto of leaving something behind. What about the hospital you're building in Kabul? How did you come up with the idea to build it and where does it fit into La Chaîne's overall mission?"

"Originally we had no plans to build a hospital in Afghanistan," Eric said. "That was the brainchild of Marine Jacquemin."

That was another name not familiar to me. "And who is Marine Jacquemin?" I asked.

They said she was a well-known French war correspondent and TV journalist who had covered news in Afghanistan for twenty years. Jacquemin was in Kabul in 1996, during the early days of the Taliban. An Afghan doctor she knew, a political opponent of the Taliban, took her to the site of the old Aliabad Hospital. It had been destroyed and the grounds around it were littered with rockets and tanks. That would have been the same hospital I saw just a few days earlier. The ground was no longer littered with rockets and tanks by the time I saw it but, otherwise, the building must have looked at least as bad as it did in 1996.

The doctor expressed his hope to Jacquemin that someday the French would rebuild Aliabad Hospital. There was some basis for his hope. The French had a long history of involvement with it. French doctors taught in Kabul's Medical University before World War II. The relationship was expanded to include French mission teams coming to Kabul and Afghan trainees going to France after the war. In the 1960s, the French government carried out an extensive rehabilitation of the Aliabad Hospital.

Jacquemin left Kabul and didn't return until November 2001, after the fall of the Taliban. When she returned she discovered that the doctor who had dreamed the French would rebuild the Aliabad hospital had been hung by the Taliban. She was deeply affected by this tragedy and returned to Paris committed to fulfill his dream. She approached her friend Françoise Monard at La Chaîne. La Chaîne had already built hospitals in Mozambique and Cambodia and she hoped the organization could be persuaded to build a mother and child hospital in Afghanistan. At first the people she met with were hesitant, but Jacquemin was persistent and persuaded Eric and Françoise to accompany her to Kabul, to see the need firsthand.

In Kabul they visited several public hospitals. "They were in atrocious condition," Eric recalled. "We visited Indira Gandhi Hospital. It was one of the most important sites in the country to care for Afghan mothers and children. Its condition was a real shock for us. It was practically destroyed. It was so dirty, with no windows and no heating. It would have been a major project to rebuild or refurbish it."

They were convinced of the need for a high quality hospital. They were also convinced that La Chaîne would have to build a new hospital rather than trying to rehabilitate an existing one. They arranged a meeting with President Karzai. He was supportive and without hesitation committed land for construction of a hospital at the Kabul Medical University campus, adjacent to the old Aliabad Hospital, exactly the site Jacquemin visited with the doctor in 1996.

La Chaîne began fundraising in France. Madame Chirac, the First Lady of France, visited Kabul in May 2003 and laid the hospital cornerstone. By July 2004, the necessary money for construction was raised and Bouygues began construction. "I realized that was just the beginning," Eric said. "Now we had to figure out how to manage the place. This project would be more than we could handle ourselves."

The La Chaîne team expanded on the information I had been given by Bouygues' representatives in Kabul. They explained how they intended to operate the hospital when it was completed.

Volunteers were the centerpiece of their plan for staffing the hospital and for training Afghans. The hospital had been planned by a Paris-based mix of salaried staff, consultants, and volunteers. Teams of volunteers would conduct on-site missions to perform surgeries and to train Afghan surgeons, nurses, and other staff. They emphasized that French volunteers would be an ongoing, long-term contribution to the hospital.

They discovered that finding a partner to operate a hospital in Kabul wasn't going to be easy. Before approaching the AKDN they had been in touch with possible partners in French-speaking Canada, with Médecins Sans Frontières and Médecins du Monde, and with the Bill Gates Foundation. None of them were interested.

I was impressed by their passion for the project. Their approach seemed both convoluted and artful. I wondered, however, how the AKDN might fit into a picture that was already substantially drawn. They assured me they were open and flexible to the nature of a partnership with the AKDN, but they would be steadfast on two points – their commitment to the hospital's philanthropic mission and its focus on women and children.

The consequences of involvement with this project would be major for the AKDN. Operating a high quality hospital in Kabul was a daunting undertaking. Security was obviously an issue but that was just the start. How could skilled nurses, doctors, technicians, and other necessary staff be trained or recruited? Afghans were one of the poorest populations in the world. Who could pay for high quality care? How could the hospital have sufficient resources to provide an international standard of care when so few patients had any ability to pay? Who would carry the financial burden of that? Would the founding partners have to shoulder the cost of it indefinitely?

The AKDN had decades of experience delivering high quality services to some of the world's poorest populations in Pakistan, India, Central Asia, and East Africa. Enormous amounts of the Network's own resources underwrite the costs of those services. While the Network is a charitable enterprise, it operates under two important principles. First, those who can afford to pay the full costs of services should do so and, to the extent possible, everyone should pay something, at whatever level they can. This approach instills a sense of ownership and respect for the value of services and upholds individuals' dignity. A second principle is that AKDN hospitals all operate as private, not-for-profit entities. That doesn't mean financial surpluses aren't pursued. They are, but any surplus remaining after collecting income and paying expenses is reinvested in the hospitals. No individuals or outside parties profit or gain from proceeds of AKDN hospitals.

Both La Chaîne and the French government had considerable emotional and financial stake in the hospital. It was not likely they would hand over responsibility to another party and fade into the background, nor should they. I was convinced that La Chaîne and the AKDN shared many positive qualities, not the least of which was passion and commitment to serve the interests of Afghan mothers and children. With that as a base, hopefully the rest could be worked out. I thought exploring a partnership with La Chaîne was worth a try. I would recommend to my AKDN colleagues that steps be taken to pursue it.

I returned to Aiglemont after my meeting with La Chaîne. I composed my written report and left it for His Highness. I departed

France for Chattanooga on July 14. I found it interesting that I arrived in Kabul on the Fourth of July, American Independence Day, and I was departing Paris on Bastille Day, French Independence Day. I doubted if that portended anything important, but it was a curious coincidence. At least it made a good story. The whole trip had been a good story. I was introduced to a new world of interesting work in a fascinating place. I looked forward to playing a role in the story for a while longer.

THE ROAD TO
A PARTNERSHIP

When I returned home, the pace of my previously placid life in Tennessee was changed considerably. Now my days were spent developing service and business scenarios for the hospital. There were frequent international teleconferences with AKDN colleagues in France, Afghanistan, and elsewhere around the world. Occasionally our telephone in Soddy Daisy would ring and the voice on the other end would inform me that His Highness would like to speak with me, or schedule a conference call. I now hardly had time to mow the grass. I loved it.

Negotiations got underway in late 2004. They would go on for more than a year before a final Memorandum of Agreement creating the framework for the partnership was established. For the rest of that year, and into early 2005, I was frequently summoned to travel from Chattanooga to Paris for meetings. Initial negotiation sessions were held at the French Foreign Ministry headquarters on Paris's Left Bank, near the Quai d'Orsay. When Pat and I lived in Paris we were often awed, as most visitors are, by the stately and august architecture of French government buildings and national monuments. More than almost any place else in the world they whisper "Empire." The Foreign Ministry was a classic example.

During my trips to France, I would usually go first to Aiglemont to meet with other members of the negotiating team. On some occasions we flew from Aiglemont to Paris on His Highness' private helicopter. When we landed at the heliport at *Issy-les-Moulineaux*, in the southwestern suburban area of Paris, one of His Highness' cars would meet us and transport us to the Foreign Ministry. Climbing the steps of the main entrance and entering the West Entrance Hall, we were surrounded by large wall-hung tapestries, sculptures, full-length portraits of notable French diplomats, elegant chandeliers, and resplendent ceilings, all which proclaimed the grandeur of French history. Alternating my life between Tennessee and the Foreign Ministry in Paris was fascinating, but also a bit disorienting, sort of like listening to bluegrass and classical music at the same time.

Each partner organization approached the negotiations with its own expectations and reservations. La Chaîne initially thought of the AKDN more as a potential donor to assist in equipping the hospital, rather than as a full-fledged partner. The idea of partnership evolved slowly. Jean-Roch recalled, "At first it was difficult for us to understand all the branches of the AKDN. It seemed they all had initials – AKU, AKF, AKHS, AKTC . . . . We didn't know at all what the Aga Khan University was. Eventually we began to realize that all the guys sitting at the table in front of us were real professionals."

Eric admitted that even though some members of La Chaîne's team had begun to form good relationships with individuals within the AKDN, their colleagues in France were resistant to the partnership. "It was very difficult to explain to Marine Jacquemin and all the team in Paris. They were completely against it. They said 'we will lose our soul. It will become a Pakistani hospital. It will become a private clinic – and the welfare, what about the welfare?'"

The idea of a public-private partnership in the social sector was also not broadly supported within the AKDN. The Network was, for good reason, confident of its own values and standards of quality and service and it was wary of putting itself into a position to be controlled, or even substantially influenced, by others. The AKDN had its own agenda that needed to be included in a Memorandum of Agreement.

Assuming our most optimistic financial projections were even close to correct, they wouldn't convince a sharp businessman that this hospital was a good investment. But La Chaîne and the AKDN had other reasons to invest in Afghanistan. Their first and shared commitments were to reconstruction of the nation and improving the welfare of its people. They wouldn't waste precious resources, but neither would they hesitate to take on the project just because it was financially challenging. They had higher purposes in mind beyond return on investment.

While the negotiations were still underway, my life was changing in other ways. I was approached in May 2005 by Shamsh Kassim-Lakha, AKU's president, to re-join the University on a full-time basis. A few months earlier, His Highness had given AKU the responsibility to govern and manage an existing AKDN hospital in Nairobi, Kenya. For nearly fifty years that hospital had been a non-teaching community hospital, governed locally and managed by Aga Khan Health Services. His Highness wanted AKU to develop it into the premier service and teaching hospital in Sub-Saharan Africa. While AKU had an international charter, thus far it had operated only in Pakistan. Now it truly had an international mandate.

The University's leadership had to immediately consider how they would manage this important new responsibility. Shamsh contacted me and asked me to launch a new position – Vice President, Health Services. If I accepted the offer I would oversee AKU's hospital programs, which would now be operating in both Pakistan and East Africa. This would include integrating the hospital in Nairobi into the overall University structure. His proposal made sense. I had been CEO of the hospital in Karachi for six years. When I worked at Aiglemont, I served on the boards of the four Aga Khan hospitals in East Africa, including the one in Nairobi. I had extensive knowledge of the place.

The problem was that neither Pat nor I had any interest to leave the U.S. again for a long-term expatriate-living situation. It had been both difficult and expensive for us to resettle in the U.S. after our nine-year stint living abroad. Not only did we have to buy a house to live in, we had to buy clothes, furniture, automobiles, and everything else we didn't have for our new stateside life. On top of that, we were both in our sixties and the thought of living abroad again, even for a few years, seemed like it would be harder the second time than it was the first.

That being said, Pat realized that I was very excited about the challenge of the work and that I would like to be involved in some way. She knew how poorly I was coping with retirement and how much I would enjoy working again with my friends in the AKDN.

"I have no interest whatsoever in moving overseas again," she declared, "but you'd like to get involved with those guys again, wouldn't you?" I admitted that I would, but I didn't see how that could happen without it being a hardship for us.

"We'll just have to set some limits on it," she said, "and they'll have to agree to them."

After some weighty discussion we agreed that I would consider taking the job, but only for one year. During that year the University would have to recruit a replacement for me. After that, if they wished, I might consider continuing in a part-time role – but I would do so from my home in the States.

Another thing that was important was for us to be able to get together from time to time during the year, either by way of me coming home or Pat meeting me someplace overseas. We didn't think that should be a problem. There were certain to be some good international travel opportunities, at least to Paris, London, Nairobi, and probably elsewhere too.

Shamsh agreed to our conditions without hesitation. He wanted me to accept the role, but he knew Pat well, and respected us as a couple. He didn't want my work with the University to be an unpleasant experience for us.

I rejoined AKU for a one-year, full-time stint in April 2005. I was still involved in the FMIC negotiations and, shortly after starting work with the University, I had to travel from Nairobi to Paris for that purpose. I felt sure my work on the FMIC project would soon wind down and that the main focus of my job from then on would be upgrading the hospital in Nairobi and integrating it into the University. I didn't know that the work agenda I had committed to was about to become even bigger than Pakistan and East Africa. It would also include Afghanistan.

I was the only health professional with hospital operating experience involved in the project throughout all the negotiations. I was concerned that at some point, if an agreement was finally reached, some organizational entity – not just one person – was going to have to quickly get involved and take charge. I raised my concern on more than one occasion but His Highness was in no rush to commit his thoughts, or to declare his decision on the matter. As I saw it, there were really only two Network entities from which to choose: either the University, with its significant academic and management presence in Karachi, or Aga Khan Health Services, from its base in the Social Welfare Department at Aiglemont. In the near-term FMIC would not be a teaching hospital; hence, I assumed responsibility for it would be given to the Health Services. It was historically responsible for the management of AKDN's non-teaching hospitals and community health programs throughout East Africa and Pakistan, and it was already in Afghanistan.

Two months after I started work with the University, His Highness' office at Aiglemont contacted me in Nairobi and asked me to join a conference call involving Shamsh and Nadeem Khan, the director general and CEO of AKU's hospital in Karachi. His Highness informed us during that call that the University would be the AKDN's designated organization to manage FMIC. Shamsh and Nadeem were taken aback. Until then they had no clue this significant new responsibility was coming down the road. They felt the University already had its hands full with the hospital in Nairobi. Taking on management of another hospital, especially one in Afghanistan, was a daunting prospect. Nevertheless, once the assignment was made, even though negotiations with the French were still going on, they wasted no time getting involved.

Up to this point, the limited group of people involved in negotiating the Memorandum of Agreement had dealt with mainly high-level issues. Now, a different group of people had to do the hard work of translating lofty principles and goals into reality. I found myself on both ends of that continuum. That wasn't a problem for me. I was growing more charmed by the place the longer I was involved with it, and I was excited to continue my involvement with it.

I felt Nadeem would be essential to our success in Kabul. He reported to me in my capacity as vice president for health services. I had known him since I first joined AKU in 1992. For six years he was one of my key administrators and right hand man. He was responsible for administrative support to most of the hospital's clinical services, but his contributions went far beyond those areas. I promoted him to the position of chief operating officer before I left Karachi to join the staff at Aiglemont. He reported for a couple more years to another expatriate CEO until, in 2000, he became the first Pakistani national to be director general of the hospital. That was a milestone for the University and a big honor for Nadeem.

Nadeem has a great sense of humor and displays it with an unrestrained laugh. His high-pitched guffaws can often be heard throughout the administrative offices. He graduated with honors from the London School of Economics and takes great pride in the fact that he is a chartered accountant. He loves history and is a walking encyclopedia of historical events and dates. He has a photographic memory and can recall facts and data to the amazement of his coworkers. I am the first to admit that I am not a detail-oriented person. My leadership style tends toward the big picture and the vision and strategy side of things. Nadeem has an incredible knack for details and organizing work. Guys like me need guys like him.

Nadeem was excited about the prospect of working with me in Kabul. His interest in Afghanistan was more than professional. He was born in Pakistan, but his ancestry is Pathan and his family placed great emphasis on their Pathan roots. "My association with Afghanistan is deep," he explains. "Afghanistan means land of the Pathans. It is where our forefathers came from. Our family tree extends back to Afghanistan and Northwest Pakistan." He views the British-imposed *Durand Line*, which separated Pathan tribal communities in Pakistan and Afghanistan, as an artificial separation of ethnic Pathans.

Nadeem's father was an officer in the Pakistan military and was stationed in Peshawar, near the Afghan border, during much of Nadeem's youth. Nadeem often travelled from Peshawar to Kabul in the late 1960's to watch Indian movies. "In those days," he said, "Kabul was a sleepy, laid-back city with a population of about 250,000 to 300,000, compared to the present four million plus. My classmates and I used to take school party trips to Kabul. We were a co-ed school. There were about forty of us. We stayed in dormitories at Kabul University, just across the road from where FMIC is now. We were very fond of Indian films, but they were banned in Pakistan. That was a fun time in Kabul. Much has changed since then. It is a different place now."

Unfortunately, that was true. Decades of war and hatred had sucked the joy out of Afghanistan. I thought about the Daliesque cinema I saw in Kabul, the one with the stairway that spiraled upward to nowhere. Maybe Nadeem and his classmates had watched movies there. I wondered whether they climbed those stairs to sit in a balcony that no longer existed.

BUILDING
LOCAL LEADERSHIP

The administrative and clinical staff at FMIC included a blend of nationalities and cultures. They were working level realists with potentially competing value systems. Several French volunteers and La Chaîne staff were already on-site preparing to open the hospital, and some Afghan doctors, nurses, and support staff had been hired. Those relationships had started to gel. The AKU team was going to be the latecomer that had to insert itself into that milieu.

In July 2005, in consultation with Eric and Jean-Roch, Nadeem and I selected individuals from AKU in Karachi and appointed them to fill senior FMIC positions in nursing, finance and administration, and professional and support services. All were Pakistanis. We sent teams to Kabul to develop a plan for management of FMIC. During the next several weeks we assessed nearly every aspect of the organization. We developed a service rollout plan and refined our earlier budget and financial projections.

It was almost inevitable that there would be issues. French volunteers – doctors, nurses, and others – were leaving their homes and jobs in France and traveling to Afghanistan to give their time and expertise on the hospital's behalf. They were confident of their own approaches to providing quality patient care, and they were comfortable and familiar with the systems that were in use at their hospitals in France. They had a strong sense of ownership of the place. As far as they were concerned, a mother and child hospital in Kabul was the manifestation of a French vision. Funds for the place had been raised from thousands of French citizens and businesses. High ranking French personalities had been attracted to the cause, including the First Lady and prominent media personalities.

There were clashes between the French mission teams and the AKU management team from the beginning. Emotions ran high and tears were shed. You could feel the tension and sense the unstated question: "Who do these Pakistani upstarts think they are?" If relationships were not managed with sensitivity there could be real and ugly problems.

The French viewed the AKDN and AKU as being too business and goal-driven, too systems-oriented, and too policy- and strategy-focused. The AKU team thought the French approach was too loosey-goosey and *laissez-faire*, too unstructured, situational – and emotional. These characteristics, on both sides, had their strengths but, if carried out excessively, they could also have their downsides. Applied side-by-side they were potentially a toxic mix.

It was important that Eric, Jean-Roch, Nadeem, and I set the leadership tone and ensure that our respective teams were open-minded, tolerant, and cooperative with one another. The four of us often had to conduct cultural sensitivity counseling sessions. But even at our level differences in approach to work were apparent.

Like Nadeem and me, Eric and Jean-Roch are a complementary team – a sort of Yin and Yang. Eric is the fount of passion under-pinning FMIC. In a subtle way he is an *Indiana Jones*-type. He is a distinguished surgeon who, in his paid day job, runs a 60-bed cardiovascular service in a prominent teaching hospital. I'm sure he is good at that, but his other, and possibly truest, passion is to run off to arduous and sometimes unsafe places like Afghanistan. He likes drama.

Jean-Roch provides balance to Eric's passion. He is an experi-enced senior business executive. He is patient, steady, rational, and well-versed in business plans. La Chaîne recruited him to be on its board when he was still the head of Siemens' medical branch in France.

"One day these guys showed up in my office, three or four of them. I knew them. I considered them to be dreamers," Jean-Roch recalled. He did, however, accept their invitation thinking it would only require a few evenings of his time each year. A few months later they asked him to create and chair a financial committee. "Now I was spending two evenings every month with them."

The die was cast for Jean-Roch. His relationship with La Chaîne strengthened and soon he negotiated his departure from Siemens. "I left Siemens one morning and by the afternoon I was working at La Chaîne as their Treasurer." He worked first as a volunteer. Three years later he was the organization's full-time salaried chief executive officer.

Our differences in style and priorities became evident right off the bat. Nadeem and I shared the findings of the AKU team's assessment of the facility at one of our first meetings in Kabul. We proposed a plan to implement and manage the hospital's services. We thought the opportunities were many, and that much detailed work had to be done. Management systems and policies had to be developed. La Chaîne had equipped the hospital substantially with used equipment donated by French hospitals. We were concerned about its quality and the ability to maintain it and keep it operational. The hospital was well-constructed; nevertheless, there were issues and defects to be corrected.

Nadeem highlighted one important issue we thought would be easy and inexpensive to correct. "There are no provisions for curtains or screens between beds," he said. "And the windows in the consulting clinics are transparent. People can see into the examination rooms. That has to be corrected. Some of our patients will be adolescent females. They will need the utmost privacy." He also pointed out that the hospital should meet international safety standards and codes. For example, no doors in the hospital would automatically close in case of fire. That had to be corrected.

Eric expressed his dismay. "Lee, you and Nadeem come to this meeting with a lot of paper. You have an action plan that has fifty-two items on it. You say the hospital is not equipped properly. You say we have to have better curtains between beds and put film on the examination room windows so people can't see in – and special doors in case of fire! How is this possible? We just finished building this hospital and you want to change fifty-two things! It is a nightmare!" He was also intrigued and skeptical about our insistence on preparation of long-range financial forecasts. "How can you know what is going to happen in fifteen or twenty years? Nobody can know that." I admitted, to myself, that there was an element of truth to his point-of-view.

Jean-Roch saw the merit of our recommendations and how they would benefit the hospital. "You are right," he said. "Our planners overlooked these things. The issue of the curtains and the film on the windows is culturally important for Afghan females. You know these things from your experience in Pakistan. We have to get accustomed to and accept your vision on these matters."

We soon came to accept, and even enjoy, our differences in management and leadership styles. We continued to approach things differently, but our relationship was built on trust and respect for one another. Eric acknowledged that this was all different for La Chaîne because, in the past, it tended to deal with problems as they arose, often as an emergency.

He eventually expressed his view of the partnership in his characteristic picturesque and passionate style. "It is clear to me now we are very lucky to have a partner like the AKDN. It is a star in our beautiful story. Without AKDN this project would be impossible. We have to be honest, we could not do it alone. It would be necessary for us to put all the power of La Chaîne onto just this one project. We will learn a lot here – on the medical team, on human relationships. For me it is a real miracle."

Some of the most important positions to be filled were the clinical department heads. We wanted to fill all of those positions with Afghan physicians. Several of the prospects had received advanced training in France, Germany, and elsewhere, and more were scheduled to go to France for training. Others had received extensive but un-credentialed experience and training while they were refugees in Pakistan and Iran. In fact, many Afghan surgeons had more surgical trauma experience than surgeons in developed countries.

We appointed eight clinical department heads. We were pleased to be able to appoint well-qualified Afghan females as the heads of cardiology and intensive care services. Only one position, the head of the laboratory, was not assigned to an Afghan physician. There wasn't a single physician in the country with advanced training in clinical pathology. An expatriate Pakistan pathologist was recruited to fill that role.

Dr. Jalil Wardak

The life stories of FMIC's Afghan staff are diverse, but all reflect their remarkable experiences in a country beset by war. One such example is Dr. Jalil Wardak. I first met Jalil in 2005, when he was a candidate for a position in the pediatric general surgery department. Jalil is a gentleman who smiles easily and often. He is always well-groomed, but a crop of unruly hair gives him a boyish and good-humored demeanor. Despite his pleasant countenance, it is easy to see a serious and introspective side to him. His character is shaped by experiences that never lie far below the surface. I realized, when I heard his story, what a patriot he is and how deeply he cares for his country.

Jalil was born in 1969, in Wardak Province. "My parents were from there. For this reason we use it as our name." He is married and has three children, twin girls and a boy. He graduated in 1986 from one of Afghanistan's best high schools and then attended Kabul Medical University, where he graduated in 1992. That was the time when the post-Soviet Najibullah Communist regime was overthrown.

He remembers the period of the Mujahidin civil war as the worst time of his life. "In our last year at medical school we were required to do clinical work in hospitals. I worked in the Aliabad Hospital, right next door to where FMIC is now. One day we saw everybody start running and they were scared. We asked what was going on. They said 'The Mujahidin came!' After that everything changed. There were no more police or people's armies – just Mujahidin fighting one another."

After finishing medical school he joined Indira Gandhi Hospital as a junior doctor. He worked there for nine years, through the civil war and Taliban periods. I said I couldn't imagine what it must have been like to work in a hospital in Kabul during those times. I asked him to tell me about it.

"We got a lot of experience but, unfortunately, it was just in war surgery. Every day more than twenty children came into the pediatric surgery department. There were too many problems. If I told you what our conditions were you would say it is too much to believe."

"I've seen a lot of tough things in my life," I said. "Try me. Tell me about them."

"Well, there was usually no electricity and no water. There was no diesel fuel for electricity. The majority of time we operated on patients with just the small light of a laryngoscope. We never washed our hands. Water was too scarce. There was no suture material and there was no system for sterilization . . . but we were obliged to do what we had to do with what we had."

He was right. It was almost too much to believe. I had worked in operating theaters in Vietnam under some pretty primitive conditions, but nothing like what he described.

Performing surgery in Kabul wasn't only complicated by a lack of basic resources. The war often intruded on surgery. "On two or three occasions there were big attacks near where I worked. Rocket attacks happened while we had patients on the operating table. My ears were deaf for many days from the explosions. It happened many, many times. Every day there would be an explosion only 200 or 300 meters away. It got to the point where it was no longer a shock or surprise. It just became usual. It was like that until the Taliban came."

Jalil lived beyond the Kabul airport, far from the hospital where he worked. He rode to work on a bicycle. "I rode my bicycle right through the airport. There were no flights then. The airport was completely empty. Getting to work required running a gauntlet. I had to pass through different 'kingdoms' of Mujahidin parties – the party of Massoud, Dostum's army, and the people who belonged to the Hizb-i-Islami party – Hekmatyar's people.

"Did it help that you were a doctor? Did that matter to any of them?" I asked.

"Of course it did, but not in a good way. Often I would be stopped by a Mujahidin faction just because I was a doctor. They would make me perform medical duties for them. When I finished doing something for one group, I would go down the road and be stopped by another one and they would say, 'You did that for them, so you have to do this for us.' The worst part was that sometimes, while we were there, they were fighting against each other."

What a life that must have been, to have had to endure that every day. All I could offer was, "It must have been very dangerous."

"It was. Sometimes missiles were flying. I spent years like that – not only me, but many of my friends and colleagues did the same thing."

Although Jalil's parents and close relatives remained in the country during the fighting, none were injured or killed. "My father always said we had to stay here. When fathers and mothers in Afghanistan say something, that is the rule. Sometimes I wanted to leave, especially to the U.S., but we stayed through the Communists, the Mujahidin, and the Taliban. We lost a lot of our friends during the war."

Jalil discovered one kind of violence was replaced with another when Kabul fell to the Taliban in 1996. "I say honestly that when Kabul was captured by the Taliban many Afghan people were very happy. They brought flowers to the Taliban. I was also happy, but on the first day, just the very first day of their stay in Kabul, I realized they were just another kind of problem."

On the first day the Taliban occupied Kabul, it became clear what life would be like under its regime. Taliban members brutally killed Najibullah, the former head of the Communist People's Democratic Party and former president of Afghanistan. Najibullah lost his support to stay in power when the Soviet Union collapsed in 1992. He tried to leave the country but was blocked from doing so, and he sought asylum in the Kabul United Nations compound. Mujahidin fighting intensified after his regime's fall, but he remained safely at the UN compound for the next four years. He was there when the Taliban came for him on September 27th. They castrated him and then dragged him to death behind a truck. For good measure and for everybody to see, they hung him from a traffic light alongside his brother who had been his security guard in the UN compound.

Jalil was on duty at the hospital when he heard of Najibullah's fate. "I heard on the radio that they killed Dr. Najibullah. It was a bad moment for me. I liked him. No one in my family was ever in the Communist party – never, but when he was president I completed my education. I had great opportunity during his reign and Kabul was very beautiful and nice at that time. I was upset and sad when I heard the Taliban hanged him. Even today when I recall it I am sad. If he was a criminal he deserved to be tried for his crimes. Of course he made a lot of mistakes. I know that. But for me, the way the Taliban killed him was criminal. Islam is a religion that gives everybody an opportunity to defend themselves. Everybody deserves to be able to defend themselves. This is the rule everywhere, in all religions all over the world."

Life in Kabul under the Taliban quickly became complicated. In one sense it was almost peaceful but, in another, the city became, in Jalil's words, "strangulated." "They stopped music and TV, a lot of things that are important for life. I am religious. I go to mosque. I pray. I like traditional clothes, but I don't like to wear them always – and I like beards, but not too much. When something becomes obligatory Afghans don't like that. I think everyone feels the same, including Americans, but in my understanding Afghans are more like that. It was too much. You had to have beards and wear turbans."

Jalil didn't escape Taliban "punishment," but his incident of punishment had an ironic twist. "Sometimes they stopped people on the street and forcibly cut their hair. It happened to me once and I was shocked. My hair was not too long. I don't like it too long. The man who did it to me . . . the one who cut my hair . . . later his own child was injured. Then he came to me and wanted to apologize so I would treat his child. I did, but it was too late for his apology. It didn't mean anything to me. The situation had changed."

Jalil said that while the Soviet health system didn't always conform with Afghan society and culture, at least under the Soviets a system existed. "During the war everything was destroyed. There were no training programs and a lot of doctors and surgeons left the country. A lot of my classmates, very clever people, are doing well in other countries now. I know they help people there, but I think our people in Afghanistan need more help than those countries do."

The 9/11 attacks and the U.S.-led invasion of Afghanistan to overthrow the Taliban and Al-Qaida brought new hope to Jalil and his colleagues.

"All the people were very happy because we had new hope for our lives, our children and for our families. During the Mujahidin and Taliban everything was stopped and there was no hope for the future. After the Taliban were driven out things were different. Before, all the doors to Afghanistan had been closed. Suddenly they were opened. Many people, including me, found opportunity to connect with health systems in other countries."

Jalil's life immediately changed for the better. His government sent him to Italy for training. "It was my first trip ever outside Afghanistan and it was to a beautiful country. I spent four months at a big hospital for children in Florence. I was pleased to be there, but I was sad because I saw how much difference there was between our system and theirs. But now we had the opportunity to change."

Jalil learned about FMIC while the hospital was still under construction. He heard it would be modern and well-equipped and without hesitation he submitted his curriculum vitae to the committee interviewing surgeons to work in it. He and one other surgeon were selected to fill positions in the general pediatric surgery department. Both were sent to France for additional training, with funds provided by the French government. Jalil was appointed as the department head.

We had two other important senior management positions to fill – the medical director and the hospital general director, or chief executive officer. Before AKU assumed management of the hospital, La Chaîne had already identified individuals to fill those positions. It was important that Nadeem and I agree to their appointments. If AKU was going to sufficiently exert its management influence on FMIC, the medical director and general director would be critical agents in its behalf. Their management capabilities and their fit with the University's values mattered a great deal.

We saw the medical director as being the essential person to oversee clinical practice and to ensure the highest standards of clinical quality. The quality of care would be the factor that most defined FMIC's long-term success and its reputation. We respected the commitment to quality demonstrated by La Chaîne – and by its surgical and medical mission teams; however, we felt it was important to bring AKU's influence to bear on that as well. La Chaîne saw the medical director as its onsite agent, communicating back to the organization in Paris and coordinating visits of the French mission teams. In its eyes, the person filling the position was critical to maintain the good will and morale of the dozens of French citizens who would travel from academic centers all around France in order to work in Kabul.

Dr. Alexander Leis

The person La Chaîne chose to fill the medical director position, Dr. Alexander Leis, didn't quite fit a traditional mold. He was born in Germany, but he attended medical school and received his pediatric training in France. His family was culturally and religiously diverse. His mother's family was from democratic West Germany and was Catholic. His father's family was from Communist East Germany and was Protestant.

Alex received his education through the Catholic Church but he was also schooled in the Protestant ethic that only hard work achieves salvation. He told me his family's experiences during World War II shaped the lessons they imparted to him. "I was taught that whatever you have, you must share. I think because of those influences I became a doctor."

In France he was a fast-rising star. He was offered the opportunity to head the pediatric department at his hospital in Paris within just a year after completing his specialty training. "I could have had security in my life until retirement, but it was too early for me to make that kind of decision. I decided to do what my parents taught me, to share my experiences with people who had less than me."

How could he do that? In his mind it was easy. He turned down the offer, resigned his position in Paris and went to Africa, where he took a medical position at a hospital in Mozambique. To say he left his mark there is an understatement. He adopted an infant boy who was orphaned when his mother died giving birth at Alex's hospital. He assumed responsibility for a young woman, another orphan, who he had engaged as the caregiver for the boy at his home. Then he invited the girl's sister and her four small children to live in his house.

"Suddenly I had a family," he said with obvious pride. "I was comfortable with my life in Mozambique. I enjoyed my work at the hospital and I was teaching at the local university."

Then, one day in 2004, he was visited by a professor from Paris. The professor was working with La Chaîne at its heart center in Maputo, Mozambique. He had heard about Alex and specifically sought him out. "He told me La Chaîne had just built a new children's hospital in Kabul, Afghanistan and they wanted the quality of care there to be the same level as care in Paris," Alex said.

"We need somebody who understands what that means," he informed Alex, "but we also need someone who knows how to deal with scarcity and hardship."

"He told me I had to think about my future and he thought I should join them. I said, 'Kabul – Oh là là!'"

Alex knew about La Chaîne from the time that he lived in France. He also knew of Eric Cheysson and Alain Deloche by reputation and he respected them. "I was hesitant, but I decided to go to Paris to discuss the opportunity. That was all it took. Eric is a very convincing person. He talked me into joining them. I came back to Mozambique and told my hospital I would leave."

All of this happened very fast and Alex had to consider the welfare of his Mozambique family. Before leaving he bought a plot of land and during the next year, while working in Kabul, he directed the construction of two houses in Mozambique. "Now everything was settled. We had two houses and a piece of land."

But Alex's legacy wasn't yet complete. With his family in Germany he established a foundation to support the hospital and an orphanage. His personal journey to FMIC left a clear trail through Mozambique.

Nadeem and I did not hesitate to accept Alex's appointment as medical director. His character, his personal initiative, and his value system were all outstanding. We realized he did not have the requisite technical management experience AKU expected of a medical director, but we could work with him to fill in that shortcoming. He was an excellent pediatrician and his presence at FMIC would add immensely to its quality of care. With La Chaîne's agreement we sent him to Karachi for training in management of clinical quality programs and other important responsibilities we expected a hospital medical director to carry out.

Alex later told me how much he appreciated that opportunity to expand his knowledge. "I came to understand the logic and importance of quality management and credentialing systems, setting goals, and budgeting. We didn't even do many of those things yet in Europe. We were ahead at FMIC."

Kate Rowlands

From AKU's perspective the most critical administrative position was that of the general director, the hospital's chief executive officer. That person would oversee every aspect of operations including not only administrative, but also clinical performance. The incumbent in this role would report directly to Nadeem. La Chaîne had already hired Kate Rowlands to run the hospital. If Nadeem and I didn't agree that she should be retained, it would be a potentially contentious issue. We felt we should spend a lot of time getting to know Kate – what her strengths and weaknesses were – and what made her tick. That wasn't quite as easy as it might sound.

Kate was born in Liverpool and raised in North Wales. She is a slender, fair-skinned, chain smoker. She is never at ease in a conversation about herself and she is almost loathe to admit her accomplishments. She can easily give one the impression that she has never done anything deserving of recognition in her life. What a mistake that would be. Tracking her life and career through their chaotic and dangerous settings is like riding a bobsled.

Kate's life in the United Kingdom started in a conventional way. Her father was an anesthesiologist and her mother was a nurse, so it made sense she would choose a career in nursing. "Early in my career I did nursing in various specialties and at various places in the U.K. I thought I would be a nurse, get married, and have kids. I never thought I would follow the paths I have taken in life."

She was working in London when she was approached by a couple of her nurse friends who said, "We are going to work in the Middle East. Why don't you come with us?"

I asked her what she thought about that. "That would be quite a change, not only in your career, but in your life, wouldn't it?"

"Yes, it would be, but I didn't even think about it. I said 'Sure, why not'."

Where had I heard that statement before? Oh, I remember. That was my answer when I was asked if I wanted to go to Afghanistan.

Kate was offered a job in Bahrain, in an oil industry hospital. "It was a nice lifestyle. I liked the trappings of life and the security it gave me, but I was turned off by the level of wealth in the country and by the people I was dealing with. I went along with it for a while but I thought it was terrible."

She only stayed there a year. I asked why such a short time. She said, "I had been there a year when the Ethiopian famine started. A friend I was working with said, 'I'm going to Ethiopia. Come with me.' I said 'Where's Ethiopia?' I thought about it for a while, but not too long. I left my nice little swimming pool and the good life and took myself off to Ethiopia. Within a month I was living in the middle of nowhere, high up on a mountain, in a tent."

That experience started Kate on a life-long path of astonishing experiences caring for civilians in humanitarian and war-torn settings. She was in Cambodia during the 1997 coup and in Iraq during the Iraqi-Kurdish civil war. She was back in Iraq again during *Operation Iraqi Freedom*. She wasn't always politically discrete about where she worked. She was in Ethiopia during its famine and then in Eritrea during its war with Ethiopia. She just went where she thought she might be needed.

Kate was an old hand in Afghanistan by the time I met her in 2005. Her first foray there was in the early nineties when she worked as a surgical nurse in an International Committee of the Red Cross (ICRC) hospital. Her recollection of that period is vivid: "I came in January 1991. It was still the post-Soviet Najibullah Communist era. It was a strange world. Things were chaos. The city was under bombardment and there were many casualties. "

It got even worse after Najibullah was overthrown. In April 1992 the Mujahidin entered the city. "After that it was horrific. People were trying to continue their lives while dealing with daily bombardments. The Mujahidin were all over the city. It was awful. People went missing. At our hospital the staff wouldn't show up for work and we would wait and wait for them – and they never arrived."

Conditions got so bad the Red Cross decided to evacuate some of its staff, but to keep the hospital working with less staff. "They only gave us a couple of hours. They just said 'go'." It was a terrible experience to leave the hospital. As usual it was filled with patients. Everybody was despondent."

Kate and her coworkers left Kabul by road. They were going to Pakistan, on roads that hadn't been maintained for years. "We had to get safe passage to Peshawar through different fighting factions. We managed to do that, but we didn't know what to expect when we left one militia group and came to the next one. And all the time our minds were back at the hospital with our people. It was a very important time in my life – to be in that place then."

Kate jumped out of the Afghanistan frying pan into a Northern Kenya fire. She went there to work with Sudanese war wounded. She stayed in Kenya about fifteen months and then went home for a few months. That was short-lived. In 1994 the Rwandan genocide began, and she went there as a surgical nurse at an ICRC hospital. The hospital had been set up in a convent.

"It was the first and last time I ever slept in a convent. I had my own little nun's stall," Kate said.

I asked her to tell me about her experience in Rwanda. "It must have been dreadful being there then – and dangerous."

"When I arrived in Kigali there were bodies all over the place. It was a different type of violence than Afghanistan, but violence is violence. You can't compare violence. It was such a graphic thing to see. You're going along the road in your vehicle and look out the window . . . . God, it stunk! It's unbelievable to see people being killed in such a way. I would be lying if I didn't say . . . . I've been pretty shocked in Kabul, but it was so graphic in Rwanda," she said.

The situation was chaotic. Kate had hardly arrived when a militia started hitting her hospital with rockets. "We were still unpacking supplies from boxes. There were boxes in the ward. I'll never forget one poor little Rwandan nurse. After all she'd seen, when all the rockets started coming in she was terrified – absolutely terrified. She started screaming – and what she did – I just thought about the innocence of it, really – she just jumped into a big box. This little nurse was so terrified she jumped in this big box, crouched down and closed the lid over herself. I thought how innocent. She thought the cardboard box would protect her. It took a lot to get her out of it."

After Kate left Rwanda she went home to Wales again. She thought she should settle down for a while but, before long, she was enticed back to international humanitarian work by the newly formed organization, *Emergency Life Support for Civilian War Victims* – simply called *Emergency*. For the next few years she worked with the organization, alternating between conflicts in Northern Iraq and Cambodia.

La Chaîne recruited Kate to work at FMIC in early 2005. By then she had been back in Afghanistan for more than five years – through the Taliban era and the period after the U.S.-led coalition drove them out of power in 2001.

Emergency asked Kate to start its first operations in Afghanistan in early 1999. "We initially went into the Panjshir Valley," she said, describing that experience. "It was one of the last strongholds of the Northern Alliance. There were so many people there with no hospital before we arrived. We opened first aid posts on the front lines of combat."

Emergency decided it couldn't just operate in the northern areas and that it should also have a hospital in Kabul. As its Program Coordinator, Kate's first job was to negotiate with the Taliban. "It didn't work in the beginning. The Taliban said 'no way' . . . you know, British passport holder, woman, and all that. But my guys at Emergency said if the Taliban didn't let me come, there wouldn't be any negotiations. So they relented and I came. I found two staff that worked with me ten years before. My first office was in a mini-bus. I used to sit in the back with my scarf around my head and the two guys would sit in the front acting like they had nothing to do with me."

Emergency finally managed to build a hospital in the middle of the city and Kate took charge of it. "It wasn't the easiest time. I remember an appointment I had with the Taliban Minister of Defense. I was told that because I was a woman I wouldn't be able to meet with him face to face. He would only meet with me if I was behind a curtain. So there he was on one side and I was on the other side. It was surreal. I think my greatest compliment came when I met the Minister of Economy. He was quite high-powered and was known to be very difficult. I got up late that morning and I didn't have time to put on any makeup. I put a bag of a dress on – it looked like a tent – and my scarf. I was sitting opposite him and he said to me, 'I want to tell you something, (I thought, oh God, what's coming now?) you are the best western woman I have met (I thought, uh oh!) because you cover yourself like you should and you don't wear all that paint on yourself.' So, that was my high point."

There were occasions when the 'religious police' came into Kate's hospital and beat both Afghan nationals and the international staff with whips. "I tried to stop them, but they wouldn't stop. One time they chucked some of our Afghan staff into Toyotas and drove away with them. It took ten days to find them and get them back."

In order to ensure the safety of its staff and patients, Emergency decided to shut down its Kabul operations until it had an agreement with the Taliban. They moved operations back to the Panjshir Valley while negotiating with the Taliban. Kate went home to Wales and was there on September 9, 2001, when she heard the Taliban had assassinated Ahmad Shah Massoud, the hero of the Northern Alliance. Then on September 11, the World Trade Center was attacked.

"Everything changed. My nurses called me in Wales and said we had to get back to Afghanistan because the shit was going to hit the fan."

Mullah Omar, ruler of the Taliban, started closing borders and expelling foreigners. Kate and some members of her medical team managed to ride into Afghanistan on horseback from Chitral, in Northern Pakistan. "When we arrived back in the Panjshir everybody there was in shock over the killing of Massoud. There was a sense of doom everywhere."

Events take strange turns in war. The Taliban contacted Emergency without any further negotiations and requested it return to Kabul and re-open the hospital. Emergency's board felt the organization had to go back to give assistance to the Kabul population during this very bad time. Arrangements were made between the Taliban and the Northern Alliance for Kate, two surgeons, and two nurses to have safe passage through the no man's land between the two forces.

"By now the Americans had started bombing with B-52s. That was the worst part of the whole trip. We finally got to Kabul safely and it was wonderful to see the hospital staff again, but they were in shock. They had been through a horrific time with the Taliban and now, on top of that, they were being bombed."

Kate remembers the last days before the fall of the Taliban in vivid detail. "You could feel something in the air. It was obvious they were preparing to evacuate, but there was still the pretense that business was going on as usual."

She had a meeting with the Minister of Health. He had a reputation as being unpleasant. When she arrived he was sitting with his father on the steps of the Ministry building. They had suitcases with them. "I thought, okay, what's going on here? For the first time ever he was really lovely to me. He said, 'Hi Kate, how are you.' I would have been an idiot to not see what was going on, but we both pretended nothing was wrong. I said I had some papers and needed his signature. We could leave them and if his secretary would call us we would pick them up in the next couple of days. Everybody was playing this charade. All the while he was sitting on the steps of the Ministry with his suitcases. It's weird, but it's true."

Conditions at the hospital were precarious. "We felt like we were in a state of limbo. We didn't know what was going to happen. There were guys of many different nationalities, with weapons, all around us. They could turn on us at any time. The Afghans were speculating when the Northern Alliance would arrive . . . 'Will they arrive . . . When they will arrive?' At that time the Americans weren't going to take the city. They were just bombing. 'When will *somebody* arrive and take over?'"

Suddenly, one afternoon and night there was no movement in the city. "You could hear a pin drop. The tension was incredible. We were all inside the hospital just trying to do our work."

All hell broke loose when night fell. "Our driver, bless him, ran in to the hospital with Taliban chasing him. He was running hell-bent for leather. I tried to tell him not to run because I was afraid they would shoot him. He ran up all out of breath and said, 'They want to take the car. They want to take the car.' He had the keys tight in his fist. He wanted to protect the hospital. The Taliban looked intimidating. I said 'Come on, come . . . .' and I opened his hand and took the keys. I told the Taliban 'Take the car, no problem, take all of them.' They took the vehicle and left without any violence. They said they had to take a sick relative to another hospital. That was bullshit, but I said, 'Oh, okay. God bless you.'"

As darkness fell the staff closed the hospital gate. "All of a sudden we started hearing all the noise from the vehicles that were leaving. It went from being able to hear a pin drop to God only knows how much noise. It was chaotic! Vehicles were passing by from different parts of the city. There were armored cars. They were taking cars, any vehicle, wherever they could get them. They were breaking into them. We all knew what was happening. I have to say that the Afghan staff needed mettle and courage because we knew if the Taliban decided to break in, the Afghans would catch hell for staying with us. They would have been the first to go."

Throughout the night the hospital staff could hear all the different languages being spoken outside their locked gate. "We could hear Uzbek, Kyrgyz, and God only knew what else. It was bedlam, some of them banged on the gate. They knew we were there but they left us alone. They had nothing to lose, but apart from taking the car they didn't harm us."

The next morning the change in the city was incredible. "At about 5 a.m. we could hear the city waking up. The Northern Alliance had come down to the city. It was like a chapter from history. People were coming out of their houses. They were happy. It was like a fun day, like a wedding. It was an incredible twenty-four hours. Some Taliban had been left behind, or hadn't been able to get onto a vehicle. I know that people . . . after all the cruelty . . . they weren't very tolerant toward the Taliban who were left behind. Soon patients started arriving and we just started to work like business as usual."

So that was Kate. Her story left me speechless – and breathless. As Program Coordinator for Emergency in Afghanistan she oversaw a staff of thirty expatriates and 1,000 Afghan nationals. She was responsible for the operations of twenty-five first aid posts and five 100-bed emergency surgical centers for war victims in Kabul, the Panjshir Valley, and Lashkar Gah. She ran a prison program in eight regions emphasizing medical care and human rights issues, and she ran a social program for Afghan women. If there was ever an individual who fit the mold of La Chaîne, it was Kate. She is a bona fide hero in the best tradition of La Chaîne, Médecins Sans Frontières, and Médecins du Monde. In 2002, for her dedication to humanitarian causes, she was awarded the honor *Member of the Order of the British Empire* (MBE) for her services to nursing and public health in war-torn countries. Typical of Kate, she didn't get around to returning to Britain to receive the award until 2006.

But after all that, could she prepare a budget? AKU is, after all, known for its management expertise and discipline. Would Kate be able to not only fit into the AKU model, but to provide leadership within it? Nadeem and I pondered that, but only briefly. It looked like a no-brainer to us. Kate already had a good relationship with La Chaîne and could help us build bridges with it. Perhaps more importantly, there was no chance we could recruit somebody else with her Kabul street smarts. We thought there was little we would face in Kabul that she didn't have experience dealing with. It was unlikely we could import anybody who would even come close to having her knowledge of the local scene. We were firm in our decision. Kate would be our CEO. We would compensate for whatever management shortcoming she might have by building a support staff around her.

But the decision wasn't just ours to make. Kate wasn't sure she wanted the job. In fact she was pretty sure she didn't. Nadeem and I had to recruit her to stay. Her professional life up to that point had been spent working in humanitarian situations. In those settings budgets and continuity of programs were far less important than immediately saving lives and reducing disability. She had never worked with an organization that wasn't donor supported and had to think about its own financial sustainability. She told us, "I'm afraid I won't fit the glove and the glove won't fit me."

I finally made the argument to her that persuaded her to stay and work with us. "Kate, you have devoted a good part of your life to caring for people in great need. Now you have an opportunity to go beyond the emergency and humanitarian work you have done and apply your incredible skills to a longer-term vision – one of human and institutional capacity building – for people and a nation you obviously care deeply about."

She decided it was worth a try. She accepted the general director position for a period of one year on the basis that we would all step back and take stock after that to see how it was working out.

AN INAUGURATION

It was early 2006 when the partners finally reached agreement on the terms for their collaboration at FMIC. On April 8, the hospital was formally inaugurated at a ceremony in Kabul. Representatives of the Governments of Afghanistan and France and the two private sector organizations, La Chaîne de l'Espoir and the AKDN, signed a formal Memorandum of Agreement setting forth the terms of their partnership.

Planning had been underway for weeks. It was a high profile event. The guests of honor were President Karzai, Madame Chirac, and His Highness. Other notable attendees were Dr. Sighatullah Mojadidi, the first president of the Islamic State of Afghanistan after the fall of the Communist regime in 1992; Ministers of the Governments of Afghanistan and France; and Ambassadors and diplomatic representatives from Asia, Europe, and North America. Representatives also attended from the United Nations Children's Fund (UNICEF), the United Nations Development Program (UNDP), and the media – lots of media.

Nadeem and I traveled to Kabul from Karachi a few days before the inauguration. We wanted to ensure that all last minute details were being well-handled, and to do whatever we could to help Kate operate the hospital under what we expected would be trying and demanding circumstances. Even though the partners' negotiations had been ongoing up to the last minute before the ceremony, FMIC had been open for business and providing care to patients for nearly six months.

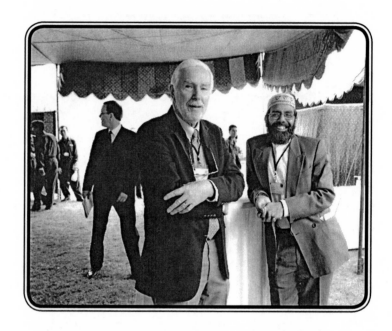

Lee and Nadeem at FMIC's Inauguration

When we arrived we found security personnel crawling all over the place. Teams from the Afghan army and the Presidential Palace were giving everybody orders and directions about how things had to be handled for President Karzai's security. French security forces were casing the place in the interest of safety for their president's wife, and AKDN security was looking after the interests of His Highness.

We found Kate in her office. She was meeting with her management team while being constantly interrupted by one security commander or another and by dozens of other visitors who all felt they required her attention to handle some detail or another.

"Lee and Nadeem!" she exclaimed. "God I am glad to see you! It's been non-stop for days."

"How are you doing, Kate?" Nadeem asked. "The place looks like a madhouse."

"Well it is," she exclaimed. "Nobody seems to know that we're trying to run a hospital here." She assured us that she and her management team were holding up and that patients were being well-cared for. "I am ecstatic that Aly Mawji's team is on top of things. It would be impossible if it weren't for him."

Aly Mawji was His Highness' diplomatic representative in Afghanistan. He had taken charge of the logistics and extensive planning of the ceremony. This was no small job. The program had to be timed down to the minute. Who would arrive when? Who would be in greeting parties? Who would participate in tours of the hospital after the ceremony? As important as anything – how would the expected hoard of aides, assistants, security personnel, press, and hangers-on be controlled?

La Chaîne representatives and French dignitaries had already arrived. Members of the French press were in the hospital taking pictures and commandeering volunteers and staff for interviews. Françoise Monard, La Chaîne's vice president, was doing her best to keep the French media under control but, inevitably, Kate's involvement was required. She had to chase after them and ensure they didn't disrupt patient care.

Managing the rest of the media was also difficult. Coverage by both Afghan and international news agencies was expected. International organizations included Agence France-Press, BBC, Voice of America, the Associated Press, Al-Jazeera, and Xinhua (China). Coverage languages included Dari, Pashto, French, English, Chinese, and Uzbek.

A potentially serious mishap occurred the afternoon we arrived. While I was walking along an outer corridor of the hospital, I looked down on the evolving scene from a second floor window. The large shamiana that would house the dignitaries and guests was already in place and erect. The center and side poles were upright and the canvas was anchored to the ground with dozens of stakes. Chairs and equipment were already in position. Everything seemed to be moving along according to plan.

The weather that day was unsettled with frequent turbulent wind gusts. While I looked out the window, as if timed just for me to see, a strong wind suddenly swept down from the mountains and picked the shamiana up, yanking all the anchors from the ground and toppling the poles. The canvas floated upward, like a giant jellyfish, to about my eye level – lines and spikes dangling below – and then it flopped, pancake-like, to the ground. I watched in dismay. Beneath the collapsed canvas I could see bulges and outlines of chairs, tables, and the dais. Very important dignitaries would be sitting and standing under there in a couple of days.

I ran down the stairs and outside. Wind and dust were swirling around the area. Several workers and some of Aly Mawji's staff were standing beside the collapsed canvas. "Is anybody hurt," I shouted.

They assured me that as far as they knew nobody was under the shamiana and nobody was hurt. We managed to get it lifted enough to see if any equipment had been damaged. Fortunately none was.

We immediately critiqued what had happened and decided that extra measures should be taken to secure the shamiana in case of inclement weather on the day of the ceremony. It was our good fortune to learn that lesson with so little consequence. What a disaster it would have been if it had collapsed during the ceremony, with all the VIPs in place underneath it!

Madame Chirac came to the hospital for a tour on the day prior to the inauguration ceremony. Nadeem was in her greeting party. He is a very devout religious person. Based on his beliefs, he doesn't shake hands with women. This is sometimes awkward.

That morning he said to me, "I am very concerned about what might happen. I am afraid the First Lady will reach out to shake my hand and I will have to refuse her. At the least she will think it bad manners on my part and at most it will be a diplomatic faux pas."

Later Jean-Roch noticed his discomfort. "Nadeem, you aren't looking well today. What's wrong?"

"I have this little problem," he said, and he explained his concern. Jean-Roch grinned and said, "No problem. We'll handle it."

Nadeem was first in line to receive Madame Chirac. She stepped out of her vehicle and toward him. She started to raise her hand, until an aide whispered something in her ear, and then she lowered it. The relief on Nadeem's face was apparent. "I heard her say 'Holy man.' After that we had a great tour of the hospital. She was a very nice and kind person."

Nadeem believed Jean-Roch must have alerted somebody on Madame Chirac's staff. He was relieved that a potentially embarrassing international incident had been avoided, which could have been captured by the French press and broadcasted around the world.

The ceremony was nearly flawless, with only a few minor mishaps, and the day was a memorable one. Nearly 300 people attended the event. Children whose conditions permitted were brought from the hospital to sit on chairs and in wheelchairs in the front row. This delighted President Karzai. He spoke to every one of them and spent more time with them than was provided for on the program.

Madame Chirac spoke during the ceremony, and she recalled her visit to Afghanistan three years earlier, when she laid the hospital's foundation stone. She was delighted that FMIC would enable Afghan children to be treated in their home country by Afghan doctors – who were trained in French hospitals – and by France's best medical professionals. She said FMIC was a sign of renewed cooperation between the Franco-Afghan medical communities and symbolic of the reconstruction of Afghanistan, with the international communities' support. She appreciated the importance of the partnership between the Afghan and French states, the AKDN, and La Chaîne. "To ensure the smooth running of the establishment, a partnership is essential," she said. "The AKDN, through the Aga Khan University, with its widely recognized professional competencies, will ensure the administrative running of the hospital."

His Highness emphasized the importance of the Government of Afghanistan's participation in the partnership. He acknowledged the nation's great need for the training of men and women in the medical and para-medical fields. He expressed a vision for the FMIC. "It is clear," he said, "that we must envisage training for nurses and doctors within this Institute." He anticipated that FMIC would develop into a high-level tertiary care center offering new specialty care essential for Afghanistan.

The chief guests were all taken on a tour of the hospital after the ceremony. Once again, Nadeem was the tour guide. The place was immaculate and President Karzai was enthusiastic to see it. La Chaîne had commissioned artwork to be painted on corridor halls – Disney characters and scenes that would appeal to children of any culture and nationality. We tried to lay down the law about how many people would be allowed to tag along, especially in the critical inpatient areas. We might as well have shouted into the wind. Managing the mob of people – the President's bodyguards and hangers-on, those accompanying His Highness and the French government dignitaries, the local and international press – was nearly impossible. Everybody was constantly jostling for a privileged position to see or be seen.

The President made it clear he wanted to visit every ward and, when he was in the intensive care unit, he wanted to meet every child and parent. The procession stopped at every bed and he chatted intimately with the staff and families. The President's security head sidled up to Nadeem and said the President was running out of time, so the last ward should be skipped.

Nadeem said he would leave it up to the President. "I told him there was another ward and he said, 'I'll go to that ward.' His security men were furious. They said I had betrayed what I had agreed to. I told them I hadn't agreed to anything." In the end, the President was happy. Nadeem escaped the episode unscathed. Despite the pushing and shoving, and occasional angry exchanges on the tour, the FMIC was formally launched.

All of the partners were fully and formally onboard and FMIC was off and running. In 2006, 1,280 patients were admitted and 23,440 outpatients were treated in the clinics. FMIC quickly became recognized as the premier health facility in Kabul. French mission teams conducted thirty-three visits to FMIC during 2006 and they worked side-by-side with the Afghan medical and nursing staff in every clinical service area. While only 689 surgeries were performed, due to involvement of the surgical mission teams, they were the most complex ever performed in Afghanistan.

Clinical advances were made almost immediately. A team led by Dr. Daniel Roux performed Afghanistan's first cardiac surgery operations in March and April -- first a closed-heart procedure, and then an open-heart procedure. Dr. Roux is based in Toulouse, France. He is qualified as a cardiovascular surgeon for both adult and pediatric patients. He has performed surgical missions for La Chaîne in Cambodia, Iraq, Sri Lanka, Senegal, Gaza, and Haiti. By the end of 2006, ninety-seven cardiac surgeries were performed, forty-nine of which were closed cases and forty-eight open-heart cases.

ISMAIL AND DR. JALIL

Another area where breakthrough procedures were performed was the Pediatric General Surgery service, headed by Jalil Wardak. The case of Ismail, son of Ibrahim Akbari, is one example. When Ismail was born he suffered from esophageal atresia, a disorder of the digestive system in which the esophagus, the tube that normally carries food from the mouth to the stomach, does not develop properly. Before his surgery at FMIC, this procedure had never been successfully performed in Afghanistan.

Ismail's surgery was performed by Jalil and Dr. Jose Uroz Tristan. Jose is a pediatric general surgeon from Spain who frequently works with La Chaîne at its sites around the world. He is a partner of SMILE Train, an organization that does corrective surgery worldwide on cleft palate and lip deformities. He is also an expert in anorectal malformation, as well as thorax surgery and laparoscopy. He has worked in Europe, Africa, Canada, and the United States. Jose left his position as head of a hospital department in Las Palmas, Spain in 2005 and went to West Africa to do humanitarian work. While there, he heard about La Chaîne and FMIC and decided he wanted to be involved. He performed his first mission at FMIC within days of its inauguration in April 2006.

In March 2012, nearly six years after his surgery, I visited Ismail and his father at their home in Kabul's District 8, in the south central region of the city. I wanted to talk with them to learn what impact FMIC's services had on their lives.

I traveled through Kabul to their home the day before *Nawroz*, one of Afghanistan's biggest holidays of the year. It is always celebrated on a date coinciding with the spring equinox. The Taliban banned the celebration of Nawroz and forbade women from participating in public events and holidays. That ban wasn't apparent on this day. As I approached the center of the city on Seh Agrab Road I passed the Kabul Zoo. The zoo is one of only a couple of public places in Kabul where families can gather in a park-like atmosphere and enjoy a respite from life's stress and the uncertainty about the future. Families – men, women, and children – were lined up along the sidewalk waiting to get in. In a departure from their usually austere dress on other days of the year, the women wore brightly colored clothes and shoes. Balloon vendors were doing a brisk business and everyone appeared in buoyant spirits. A potential damper on the holiday was a security alert warning of possible suicide attacks at public gatherings. That didn't appear to have lessened anybody's enthusiasm on this holiday.

In the center of the city we drove alongside the Kabul River. In the more than seven years in which I visited Kabul, I never saw more than a trickle of water in the river bed. Usually it was bone dry, a repository of trash and a hangout for homeless people and drug addicts. During the winter of 2011-2012, Kabul had experienced record low temperatures and the heaviest snowfalls in fifteen years. On this March day, the water in the river bed was high and easily seen from the street.

As we drove south from the center of the city we passed the Ghazi National Stadium. During the Taliban era it was known as the stadium of death. In 1999, the Taliban publicly executed Zarmina, a 35-year-old mother of seven children, in the stadium. Zarmina had allegedly killed her husband but, despite being imprisoned and tortured for three years, she never admitted her guilt. The execution was staged before 30,000 spectators, mostly men. She was transported into the stadium in the back of a Toyota pick-up truck. She was dragged from the truck and forced to kneel in front of soccer goal posts, whereupon a Taliban executioner shot her in the head. The world learned of this despicable event because it was secretly recorded on a video camera and smuggled into Pakistan. It was later shown to the outside world in an award-winning British television documentary.

Thankfully, things change. In a story about the stadium in December 2011, a Reuters news article began, "Its pitch, they said, was so blood soaked that grass would not grow. For years, the only spectacles on offer at the Ghazi Stadium in the Afghan capital were executions, stonings, and mutilations by the Taliban, rulers of the country . . . ." The article continued, "On Thursday, thousands of young Afghan athletes . . . came to the stadium to celebrate its official re-opening. This time, the grass has been ripped up and replaced with bright green artificial turf, part of a U.S.-funded stadium refurbishment." Of all international projects implemented in Afghanistan, this is cited as one of the most popular.

Ismail's home is located in a residential complex alongside a lake. Ibrahim and Ismail met us at the end of their street and walked with us to their house. Ibrahim said the lake bed was usually dry but, like the Kabul River, this year it was filled with water due to the winter's excessive snowfall.

Ibrahim welcomed us into his home, and when we were seated, Ismail brought us a tray of tea and candies. Ibrahim said he is originally from Bamyan Province. He and his family are Nizari Ismailis, followers of the Aga Khan. He said that before the Taliban he had a good job working with a non-governmental organization (an NGO) that operated in Kabul and Jalalabad. After the Taliban came the NGO stopped its operations in Afghanistan. Ibrahim went to Peshawar, Pakistan, where he was able to continue working with another branch of the same NGO. He didn't return to Afghanistan until after the fall of the Taliban. Since early-2010, he had held an administrative position in the office of the Kabul-based *New York Times* correspondent.

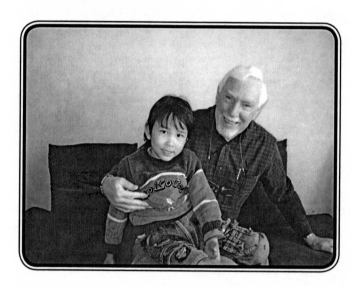

Lee Hilling and Ismail

Ibrahim apologized that his wife was not able to be with us. He explained that she was in Pakistan recovering from treatment for a serious illness. She saw several doctors in Afghanistan before finally being referred to FMIC for diagnostic studies. Doctors there found she suffered from a fungus infection, in her lungs. They told the family treatment was not possible for her in Afghanistan and she should go as soon as possible to either India or Pakistan. The family went to India, but then reconsidered and decided to go to AKU in Karachi. Doctors at AKU first recommended conservative medical treatment, but that was unsuccessful and they decided surgery would have to be done. One complete lung had to be removed. A few weeks after her surgery, her doctor said she was well enough to return to Afghanistan. Ibrahim had to return to his job but, because of the severe winter in Kabul, he felt his wife should stay in Pakistan until the weather improved. She was still there with relatives. For the time being, Ibrahim and Ismail were living alone.

Ibrahim said that after Ismail was born the family immediately realized he had a problem. "When he sucked milk from his mother's breast, instead of it going into his stomach, it went into his lungs. Everybody was telling us a different story about what we should do. Some said we should go see the Mullah at the mosque. We decided to take him to Indira Gandhi Hospital. They told us we should take him to India as soon as possible." The family couldn't do that. Ismail was a very sick newborn baby and it was unlikely he would survive such a trip.

"A friend put me in touch with a doctor who knew about FMIC," he said. "We knew it was a new hospital and had just opened. We arrived there at midnight one night. Ismail was fourteen days old. They examined him and said he should be admitted for an operation the next day."

Ibrahim knows it was the first time Ismail's kind of surgery was ever successfully performed in Afghanistan. "I am very grateful and thankful for FMIC. Ismail is very healthy now. He is six years old and he has no problem at all. If anything, he is too naughty. Now anytime he is not feeling well, for any reason, we take him back to Dr. Jalil. He loves Dr. Jalil."

Ismail hasn't yet started school. He should have started this year but, because his mother is sick and out of the country, Ibrahim decided against it. "He wants to go," he said. "He would like to study and learn to build buildings."

I thanked Ibrahim and Ismail for meeting with me and left for my trip back to FMIC. Our drive was uneventful until we reached the center of the city. Suddenly a dust storm enveloped us. The wind was intense, whipping dust and grime around us until we could hardly see the front of our vehicle. People on the street covered their mouths and eyes as they tried to continue their pre-holiday activities but, for now, the fun had gone out of the day.

We crept along the streets. As we approached an intersection near FMIC the traffic came to a stop. A motorcyclist zipped past us into the intersection while we waited in the line of traffic. A taxi blocked his way and the driver objected to him trying to pass. Words were exchanged and soon punches were thrown. A third participant joined in and a crowd gathered. What had earlier been a festive day had become a tense and ill-tempered one. This was exactly the kind of situation the security advisory said should be avoided. While everyone was preoccupied watching the fight we eased our vehicle out of the line and quietly edged our way along the street. Minutes later we arrived at FMIC.

At the hospital, I talked with Jalil and Jose about Ismail's case. Jalil told me it would have been dangerous for the family to take him to Pakistan or India, as they were advised to do at Indira Gandhi Hospital. "Patients with this condition are emergencies. If treatment is delayed the chance of dying is very high. Also, at that time, the roads from Kabul to Pakistan were completely destroyed."

Jalil said Ismail wasn't difficult to diagnose. "We learned he was born from a mother with too much amniotic fluid during her pregnancy. That is often a cause of Ismail's kind of problem. Also, he wasn't able to breastfeed and he had cyanosis and was coughing and choking. These are all symptoms of atresia. We passed a tube through his nose and it was blocked after ten to twelve centimeters. It couldn't pass into his stomach. We did an x-ray and were able to see the blockage."

An echocardiograph and sonography indicated Ismail had no cardiac complications, which can occur with esophageal atresia. Nevertheless, he wasn't stable. His lungs were full of secretions, he was dehydrated, and there was a possibility he would develop sepsis. Jalil and Jose decided he should have surgery as soon as possible.

They spent almost all night in the intensive care unit preparing for Ismail's surgery. They also had to prepare their surgery team. "This would be the first surgery of its kind at FMIC. We had to make sure the operating theater team and nursing staff were aware of the case and ready for it."

Jose said he coached Jalil but let him do most of the work by himself. "Jalil is one of the best surgeons in the world. Everything went very well. We did a very small incision and had a good approach. In the end the outcome was perfect."

The morning after surgery, Jalil told Ismail's family that the operation was successful and the recovery should be complete. The total cost of Ismail's sixteen-day hospitalization and surgery was US$744.00. FMIC's patient welfare program covered US$284.00 and the family paid US$460.00.

When Jalil worked at Indira Gandhi Hospital, he and a colleague attempted the procedure several times, but they always failed and lost the babies. "I admit that we didn't have good skill," he said. "We also lacked instruments and proper equipment. Most importantly, we didn't have an intensive care unit like we have at FMIC."

Jalil's reputation for successful treatment of esophageal atresia was well-known throughout Afghanistan by 2012, and referrals routinely came to him. Other surgeons on his staff were also able to perform the procedure. They had performed ninety-nine esophageal atresia procedures since doing Ismail's case. "When we reach the 100th case we will hold a celebration," he said. They had performed 155 esophageal atresia procedures by May 2014.

In the beginning, about fifteen percent of esophageal atresia cases performed at FMIC did not survive. This was because some had very severe congenital abnormalities, including heart disease and severe lung complications, but the main cause of mortality was late arrival at FMIC and sepsis resulting from delayed treatment.

"I recently did a case thirty-six days after birth and another twenty-eight days," Jalil said. They both survived. I think the one operated on after thirty-six days may be one of the longest after birth to survive in the whole world, not just Afghanistan. That baby was very weak, less than 2 kilograms, with lots of dehydration and sepsis."

Now Jalil and his team conduct continuous medical education sessions for doctors at other hospitals and they teach them what signs to look for when a child is born. "Now they know that when a mother has too much amniotic fluid they should anticipate this condition. We used to receive babies with esophageal atresia between seven and twenty days after birth. Now that is dramatically decreased and we often get them in the first twenty-four hours."

Sometimes referring doctors make mistakes and send patients with the wrong diagnosis. Jalil doesn't think that is a problem. "I'd rather that happened than they didn't send them to me when they should."

Jalil is convinced his decision to join FMIC was the best choice of his life. "I know I made the right choice. People in the community say 'If our children have a problem, we have FMIC.' At first it was hard. The French and AKU were bringing in new systems. Sometimes they were not acceptable for us, for example, charging patients money for their care. I had always worked in free hospitals and I thought that was the way it should be. Now I understand why it is important for a hospital to have income to replenish its resources. It is good that we have a patient welfare system to assist patients who can't afford to pay. Now I know these new systems are good for our Afghan health system. We have to change and accept other things."

Jalil's department now has five senior surgeons. They have received advanced pediatric general surgical training in several French medical teaching centers and have presented papers at French and European Pediatric Surgery Congresses. All have benefited from training imparted by mission teams from teaching centers across France. They perform a wide variety of surgical procedures not able to be performed elsewhere in Afghanistan, including laparoscopic and endoscopic, plastic, and neonatal surgeries. "We are able to provide care for almost all children's conditions except oncology," he said. "Children still have to leave the country for that."

LEADERSHIP TRANSITION

The selection of Kate as FMIC's start-up CEO proved to be a good choice. She was highly regarded by the French and held in deep esteem by the Afghans. She especially helped build strong relationships with the Afghan staff and her rapport with Afghan families was remarkable. Our anticipation of her knowledge of Kabul was correct. She knew all the major players in the city and helped build a solid relationship with the Ministry of Public Health and other Government of Afghanistan agencies.

When we recruited Kate it was done with the understanding that we would assess whether the job was a good fit for her and whether she would be interested to continue in it. By early 2007, we were moving beyond the start-up phase to one requiring refinement of FMIC's performance and development of long-term strategies, including planning for major new services and construction. We consulted with Kate and we mutually agreed that she would step down from the position. She had done the job we asked her to do. She had gotten the hospital off to a good start, but the tasks ahead increasingly required broad executive management skills.

Kate was comfortable with this. "To be honest, it wasn't the easiest time in my life. There were times when I was a nut cake, but I learned a lot of things I had never thought of before. People who knew me well questioned why I decided to work at FMIC.

I told them it was my chance to do something special. I asked them, 'Why should the Afghans only have access to poor quality medicine? Why can't they have the chance to go forward?' I was very sincere about that. Working in the hospital brought me a lot of joy. A case in point is the intensive care unit. It's incredible, not just because of the people who manage it. It's not run by international staff. It has some but it's mainly staffed by Afghan nurses and doctors. The same is true in the operating theater. I know the Afghan staff is proud to work in the hospital and to be part of it. It's not just a matter of coming to work. It's something special for them. They feel they work in a special place. I feel the same."

The good news was that Kate might continue her involvement with FMIC in another role. La Chaîne had another important job in mind for her. Jean-Roch and Eric asked her to conduct a feasibility study for a program to ensure that surgical care at FMIC would be available to the most vulnerable and poorest children from rural areas. The premise was that the only chance of survival for many children in remote provincial areas was to be treated at FMIC, but families often did not have sufficient resources to travel to Kabul. The new program would be funded by La Chaîne through donors in France and, while it would be operated independently from FMIC, it would be an extension of the hospital's patient welfare program.

The results of the feasibility study convinced La Chaîne to launch the new program and Kate agreed to head it. In March 2008, the organization opened a residential facility in Kabul to provide a home for children and their families while the children were receiving treatment at FMIC. The facility was formally named *The Children's House*, but it quickly became affectionately known as *The Kids' House*.

Kate and her team worked closely with the International Committee of the Red Cross, the International Assistance Mission, and other NGOs in Afghanistan to identify the most vulnerable children – the poorest of the poor – in remote rural areas and arrange their treatment at FMIC. All expenses, including travel for the children and their parents, their housing and subsistence at The Kids' House, and their costs for treatment at FMIC, are provided through the program.

The Kids' House is located in a quiet residential area of west Kabul, close to FMIC. It has reception and waiting areas for children and their families, and an exam room for the house nurse. Residential accommodations include a dining room, a play area and recreation room, nine bedrooms, and four bathrooms. The play room is brightly decorated with dozens of furry, stuffed animals, and assorted critters suspended from the ceiling.

At the rear of the house is a lawn surrounded by walls of flowers. Out of respect for Afghan cultural norms there are separate areas, so that men and their wives can sit on opposite sides of the lawn. In the center is a playground with swings, a roundabout, and a see-saw. A multi-colored 1970s vintage Volkswagen Beetle is parked in one corner. It's the kids' favorite play thing. They love to crawl in and out of it and pretend they are "driving."

The Kids' House is more than just a place for families to stay while the children are treated at FMIC. It is an oasis of tolerance and tranquility not commonly seen in Afghanistan. All the residents realize it is a special place, a place where the children are most important and where all their differences should be put aside. Ethnic groups mix freely – Pashtuns, Hazaras, Tajiks, Uzbeks, and more – and ethnic, political, and geographical differences are forgotten.

Kate is proud of the peaceful aura of The Kids' House. "We have ethnic groups that come from the top of the Wakhan Corridor to the Iranian border. It is touching how they all get along. They even joke about it sometimes. We've had families from the more danger-ous parts of the country and parents from other regions laughed and said 'they're dangerous.' They are not defensive or hostile to-ward one another. They discuss politics but there are no political issues. Their main concern is to take care of the children. When children need blood at the hospital parents from any ethnic group will offer to give blood to children of another group. The help of parents is completely necessary. The fathers help in all kinds of ways. The mums help with sewing, cleaning, and preparing food in the kitchen. It is wonderful. From their points-of-view, it gives them pride that they can contribute and not just take."

Kate loved her new job, and the children and parents who came to The Kids' House loved her. She once reminded me about a time when I questioned whether it was the right job for her. "When we first talked about me taking this job, you said, 'Kate, you need action, you need to do things that keep you totally occupied. It's not for you to run some small project.' You were wrong Lee. I have found great satisfaction in this job. It's not big, but the kids really benefit. It is sad that there are kids we can't help, but there are always kids we can help. Sometimes I feel a little loopy with all the emotional ups and downs, but I also feel a lot of serenity and I get a lot of pleasure out of it. I look forward to getting up and coming to work every morning."

When Kate left her position as FMIC's start-up CEO to con-duct the feasibility study, we began a search for her replacement. Within a couple of months, we had identified the ideal per-son to succeed her. Aziz Ahmad Jan was an experienced health professional with a master's degree in health management from the University of Birmingham, in the U.K. When we approached him he was working as the chief operating officer of the 550-bed Shifa International Hospital in Islamabad, Pakistan. Shifa is one of the preeminent hospitals in the region.

Aziz is an Ismaili. He was born in the remote and breathtakingly beautiful Hunza Valley, in Pakistan's Northern Area region. He is an imposing figure, both broad and tall, but his manner is gentle and good-humored. He smiles easily and often.

I interviewed him in Kabul. I asked him why he would leave a prestigious job like the one at Shifa and come to Kabul to run FMIC. "FMIC is an eighty-five bed start-up operation and it is much smaller than Shifa. Why would you even consider such a move?" I asked.

"Lee, though I am running a much larger hospital in Islamabad, I think it will be better for me to come to Afghanistan. Every day here will be a new learning experience for me. Things have more meaning here. Whatever you do here, you get important results. When we implemented CT scan or MRI at Shifa Hospital nobody noticed. I think when we do something like that here everybody will notice. It will be important."

But there was more to Aziz's motivation than that. He continued, "Besides, Lee, I have a long history working with Afghans and it means a lot to me. I ran the Aga Khan Health Service's programs in the Punjab and Northwest Frontier Provinces of Pakistan in 1990. Afghans were being terrorized and displaced by their civil war. They were pouring into Pakistan in great numbers. We set up a hospital in Peshawar to care for them."

One day, shortly after setting up the hospital, Aziz had a distressing experience. "We got a message that there had been a road traffic accident involving Afghans. We rushed to the hospital, but only one child, an eight-year-old boy, arrived. Both his hands and legs were broken. We asked 'Where are the rest of the patients?' He said his parents and brothers and sisters had all been killed. He was the only survivor. That affected me a lot – as a human being, as a father, and as a professional." Aziz remained involved with Afghan refugees for the next fifteen years. "After that, until 2005, every day and night of my life was involved with Afghan refugees."

In 2000, Aziz was appointed as general manager of all Aga Khan Health Services' operations in Karachi and in Pakistan's Baluchistan region. His duties once again involved working with Afghans. For the next five years he often worked closely with Nadeem Khan to arrange care for refugees at AKU. "There were over 100,000 refugees in Karachi at that time," he said. "It was a huge program."

His job frequently involved more than just providing medical care to the Afghans. "On many occasions Afghan women giving childbirth were at risk of dying and needed blood," he said. "Their husbands and families wouldn't consider giving blood and they wouldn't let them get donated blood either. They were afraid it would be mixed with Pakistan blood. But on many occasions they let me give blood. They accepted me as a leader, even as their brother."

Even though Aziz had worked with tens of thousands of Afghan refugees, he was never in Afghanistan until 2000. That wasn't a good experience. He was traveling with a group of other Pakistanis – doctors and health care workers – from Chitral to Peshawar.

"We were supposed to make the trip by air, but the flight was cancelled because of bad weather and we had to drive."

Normally that road trip would all be in Pakistan, but it was winter and there was heavy snow on the mountain pass near Chitral. "The mountain road was closed and we had to follow a valley road that led into Afghanistan."

It was during the Taliban time. They were able to cross several Taliban checkpoints without difficulty, but they ran into a problem near Jalalabad. "We were stopped there by Taliban guards. They all wore turbans and had long hair and beards."

One of them ordered Aziz and his group to get out of their vehicle. "Who are you? What are you doing here?" he said.

"We told him we were doctors and health care workers and we were on our way to Peshawar."

"Why do you not have beards?" another demanded.

"We told him, perhaps foolishly, that we didn't have to wear beards."

"Then you are not Muslims and you will go to Hell!"

"Then they lectured us that we should always pray when we started a trip. They asked one of our doctors, 'What prayer do you say when you start a journey?' You know Lee, we Muslims say prayers from the Koran for every part of our lives – when we eat, when we got to bed, when we travel. The doctor was very upset and said he didn't know the prayer. The Taliban said then he must be punished."

Individuals in the group who had beards were told they would be exempted from the punishment. Aziz and a dozen others who didn't have beards were led across the road. "One of them grabbed me by the shoulder and shoved me."

"Were you afraid?" I asked. "This must have been a harrowing experience. You were out in the middle of nowhere and completely under control of obviously erratic and dangerous people."

"Lee, by this time I was becoming really afraid. I thought they might kill us. But to be honest, the punishment was tolerable. They made us act like chickens. We had to squat down on the road, hold our hands over our ears and flap our arms. It literally tells us, 'You are like a cock. Get in the cock position.' We used to get this kind of punishment from teachers when we were young students in school. It is intended to be a humiliating and degrading act."

While everyone was squatting and waddling around on the road another Taliban –someone of apparent authority came on the scene. He demanded of the guards, "Why are you punishing them?" They replied, "Because they don't have beards." He was angry with them and said, "They are from Pakistan. They are our friends. Don't punish them and keep them here. Give them food and let them go."

"We were very grateful and relieved," Aziz recalled. They fed us and gave us a travel permit to show anyone if we were stopped again."

Nadeem was with me when Aziz recalled his encounter with the Taliban. He laughed and said, "After that day Aziz definitely learned the prayer you say when starting a journey. He never for-gets it."

Aziz accepted our offer and, on November 10, 2007, FMIC's board appointed him to be general director of the hospital. He was confident it would be one of the special opportunities in his life.

TEHMINA AND DR. MIRZA

The heart and soul of FMIC are the Afghan children who receive care there, their families, and the doctors and nurses who care for them. They have suffered hardships unimaginable by those privileged to live in less turbulent and dangerous places. They have courage, fortitude, and the intense will to persevere and survive in the face of adversity and danger.

Tehmina, daughter of Nazar Muhammad, had suffered from severe scoliosis, a lateral curvature of her spine, since she was an infant. It wasn't until she was thirteen years old that she finally underwent corrective surgery. Her surgery was performed at FMIC by an Afghan orthopedic surgeon, Dr. Mirza Nijrabi, and a French surgeon, Prof. Jean-François Mallet. Prof. Mallet is based at the University Hospital at Caen, in Normandy, France. He is a specialist with nearly forty years' experience treating spinal diseases. He has travelled to Kabul at least once a year since 2006 to mentor Mirza in performing spine surgery on children. I visited Tehmina and her family at their home in Kabul in September 2011.

Tehmina and her family live in Kabul's District 7, at the foot of one of the many mountains surrounding the city. They are ethnic Tajik. Afghanistan has the largest Tajik population outside their homeland country to the North. After Pashtuns, Tajiks comprise the largest ethnic group in Afghanistan. They are mostly Sunni Muslim and mainly speak Dari.

Afghanistan's most prominent Tajik, Burhanuddin Rabbani, was assassinated by a suicide bomber at his residence in Kabul just a few days before my visit. Rabbani held control of the government from 1992 until he was overthrown by the Taliban in 1996. He was the Karzai government's chief peace negotiator with the Taliban at the time of his death. The effect of his assassination on the peace process remained to be known, but it had already caused anxiety and agitation within the Tajik population.

Tehmina and Nazar Muhammad waited for me by the side of the street. Her father invited me to follow him and Tehmina through a low portal in the wall. Inside was a dirt courtyard surrounded by high mud walls. Clothes lines were strung from one side to the other. The area was dry and dusty, but the floor of the courtyard was swept clean. There was no cover overhead, so on a rainy day the area would be transformed into a slippery, muddy mess.

Steep, uneven and irregular steps curved upward to the entryway of their home. There was no handrail on the steps. I watched Tehmina climb the steps with surprising strength and balance. I followed her and entered a meticulously clean and carpeted room. Cushions lined the walls. The only furniture was a large cabinet at one end of the room. A clutter of family possessions and photographs sat atop the cabinet.

Nazar Muhammad invited me to sit on cushions on the floor. He and Tehmina sat across from me. He welcomed me to his home, expressing regret that it was so humble. Speaking through a translator I told him it was an honorable home and it was my honor to be invited into it.

Tehmina's mother entered the room with a pot of freshly brewed tea and a dish of hard candies. She poured the tea while our conversation started. We were joined by two older women who Nazar Muhammad introduced as Tehmina's grandmother and aunt. They said they lived in Pul-i-Kumri, the capital of Baghlan Province, north of Kabul. They were in Kabul for the aunt to get care for a skin disorder on her arms. She pulled up her sleeves to show me the condition on her arms. Nazar Muhammad told me that Tehmina has three brothers. The youngest, Yousuf, was introduced to me. The other two were in school.

Tehmina was fourteen years old when I visited her. She is an attractive and engaging girl, albeit a little chunkier than Mirza would like her to be, given her disability. She has sparkling eyes and a disarming smile. She was shy but not intimidated by my presence. She looked directly at me when responding to questions. In fact, she seemed pleased to be the center of attention.

I asked Nazar Muhammad when the family first became aware of Tehmina's spinal deformity.

"When she was born she had no problem," he said. "When she was six months old there was intense fighting in our neighborhood. Tehmina's mother was carrying her while fleeing for safety. She tripped and Tehmina flew from her arms landing hard on the ground. After that she had pain in her back and it just kept getting worse."

While this was undoubtedly a traumatic event for the family – and may have complicated Tehmina's condition – it likely would not have caused Tehmina's scoliosis. Scoliosis of Tehmina's type would be either congenital or acquired, due to her body's adaption to another physical malformation such as abnormal development and length of leg bones.

I asked if the family tried to get care for her. Nazar Muhammad said they had. "Her mother took her to Indira Gandhi Hospital when she was about 1½ years old."

"Were they able to do anything for her?" I asked.

"The doctor there said that if we paid 300,000 Afghanis (approximately US$6,000) they would give her a brace to wear," he responded.

I expressed surprise at that large amount of money. "Could you afford that? Did you try it?"

"No. We did not have that kind of money and there was no way we could get it. We never sought any further care for Tehmina after that."

Tehmina was left to live with the deformity and the constant pain that kept her from leading a normal life. She was unable to regularly attend school. The family feared that when she became an adult she would be housebound and require care they would be unable to give her.

Mirza had told me that, left untreated, Tehmina's future was bleak. Her deformity was certain to progress. Complications she would likely develop were neurologic dysfunction with weakening of the legs, compression of the spinal cord, contractures and limited range of motion of various joints, and respiratory problems.

After many years of living with Tehmina's condition, the family finally heard something that gave them new hope. The child of one of their neighbors had a problem that required surgery. They learned that he had surgery at FMIC and his problem was corrected. "I am unemployed and I was sure we could not afford care at such a prestigious hospital," Nazar Muhammad said. "But my neighbor said if we took Tehmina to Kate's Kids' House they would arrange for her to be treated at FMIC even if our family couldn't pay for it."

That was what the family did and Tehmina had surgery at FMIC. Nazar Muhammad says her life has been changed since the surgery. "She is no longer confined to home and she can go to school."

Tehmina was regularly attending school and was in the sixth grade. She told me that she loves school and likes all of her subjects, but that her favorite is English.

I expressed mock alarm and asked, "Have you understood what I've been saying all along? Why have I been using a translator?"

Tehmina giggled and denied that she could understand my English. All the family laughed.

"I want to go to the university and to be a doctor," she told me. "At FMIC all the doctors and nurses were kind to me. I would like to help people in my country."

As I prepared to depart, Nazar Muhammad thanked me for visiting his family. He said they will never forget the people at FMIC who cared for Tehmina. He said they have special gratitude for Kate Rowlands. "She is a special woman and is always caring for poor people," he said.

Mirza told me the procedure he and Prof. Mallet performed to straighten Tehmina's spine was called *anterior, posterior, arthrodesis and instrumentation*. Her surgery was the first time the procedure had ever been performed in Afghanistan. It entails removing intervertebral discs and the material connecting them with the vertebral body. The vertebral bodies are then connected with each other and fixed by bone from the patient's own body, usually from a rib. Arthrodesis generally involves blocking an articulation by bone fusion. The problem is that after that procedure, further growth of the child is not possible. Obviously this is not desirable. For some children, like Tehmina, the technique of instrumentation is applied. The vertebras are fixed by a metallic device, and it is possible to adjust the device after some months, allowing growth.

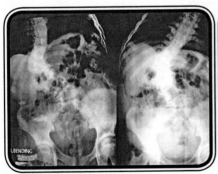
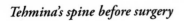
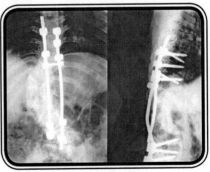

Tehmina's spine before surgery   *Tehmina's spine after surgery*

Mirza said that when FMIC opened in 2006 it was not planned that spine surgery would be done. "In the developed world, despite much better conditions than exist in Afghanistan, the complication rate for pediatric spine surgery is around forty per-cent. It was felt the rate would be even higher in Afghanistan, given all the additional difficulties to be faced, including poor nutrition and fragile bones of the children, concerns about sanita-tion and hygiene, and very advanced deformities due to failure to start treatment at an early stage."

"We began doing simple procedures," he recalled. "We finally got to the point where we could treat very sophisticated cases. We had to. A lot of patients had conditions that couldn't be treated in Afghanistan, but they also couldn't afford to travel to Pakistan or India. In the first year we saw many patients with deformation or misalignment of the hip joint. We thought we should start with this."

Mirza pointed out that in developed countries children with de-formities are identified early and their treatment is started with-out delay. This prevents the development of many complications due to delayed treatment.

"Here we see patients fifteen, sixteen, and seventeen years old – with huge deformities. We have to do something for them. At least we should prevent progression of their deformities. That is the main purpose of our surgeries."

The French mission teams have been essential to develop-ment of Mirza's surgical skills. He started doing spine surgery independently in 2008. His results have been excellent, not-withstanding the many risks involved with spine surgery in Afghanistan.

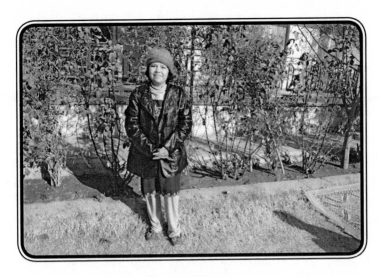

Tehmina after surgery

The total cost of Tehmina's surgery at FMIC was the Afghani equivalent of approximately US$3,700.00, much less than the proposed cost of the brace offered by the doctor at the *free* public hospital ten years earlier. In the U.S., Tehmina's hospitalization would have cost around US$80,000 to US$100,000. On top of that, surgeon's fees would be approximately US$7,000, and the cost of implants, screws, and rods, would be another US$8,000 to US$12,000.

Tehmina's family had no capacity to pay for her care. All of it was paid for by funds from Kate's *Kids' House* and FMIC's patient welfare program. Mirza says the patient welfare program is essential to FMIC's mission. "Patients cannot afford to leave Afghanistan, and the government cannot provide the type and quality of services FMIC can. We initially thought patients would not come to FMIC because of its policy that whoever has money should pay whatever they can. That hasn't been the case. Patients come to FMIC from every province. They know it gives the best care in Afghanistan."

Mirza was born in Kabul in 1960. All of his adult life has been spent in a seemingly never-ending war. His father was in the military and Mirza attended a military school for twelve years before entering medical school at Kabul Medical University. His manner and demeanor hint at his military upbringing and his later service in Afghanistan's army. He is all business. He doesn't dawdle. His conversation is to the point and he seems always ready to get on with whatever task is next. His hair and mustache would always pass military inspection.

When Mirza was in his early teens, Afghanistan's King Zahir was overthrown by his own cousin in a bloodless coup. This ended a forty-year period sometimes described as Afghanistan's golden age. During the next six years, the country went through a series of revolts, putsches, and uprisings leading to the December 1979 Soviet invasion and establishment of a Communist regime in Afghanistan.

Mirza graduated from Kabul Medical University in 1985, during the Soviet occupation, and he was assigned for three years to a military hospital in Jalalabad. That was where he got his early orthopedic experience. "We had good orthopedic surgeons," he says. "Because of the war there were many patients with orthopedic injuries and we were always very busy. There were no formal learning centers for surgery. I had books from the U.S. and some videos."

He was reassigned in 1988 to be the senior orthopedic surgeon at the National Security Hospital in Kabul. Following the Soviets' defeat, during the Mujahidin forces civil war, the National Security Hospital was sometimes the target of artillery. These were arduous times for Mirza and his colleagues. He told me the number of casualties was enormous.

"In just one day we would have more than 150 surgeries and our team sometimes had no sleep for more than twenty-four hours. During this time our health care system in Afghanistan was completely destroyed. Sometimes we had to stop patients' bleeding and do surgery without sterilization. We just did what we had to do. There were problems with blood, medicines, anesthesia, bandages . . . everything. Sometimes we had to bring in a few sutures in our pockets to use in surgeries."

The situation continued to deteriorate after the Taliban takeover of Kabul in September 1996. Many Afghan doctors and professionals fled the country during the Taliban occupation. For no good reason, the Taliban arrested one of Mirza's brothers and put him in jail for three months. When he was freed he went to Peshawar, in Pakistan. Mirza stuck it out with the Taliban for a while but he, too, was subjected to harassment and threats by them. After a few months he also took his family to Peshawar.

The migration of Afghan refugees to Pakistan began with the Soviet invasion and increased through the 1980s. According to the United Nations High Commissioner for Refugees (UNHCR) report *Searching for Solutions – 25 Years of UNHCR – Pakistan Cooperation on Afghan Refugees*, the *registered* refugee population in Pakistan peaked in 1990 at about 3,272,000. After that time, it began to decrease. Afghan refugees in Pakistan were estimated at around 1.5 million when Mirza and his family went to Peshawar in 1996. Many think these numbers are gross underestimates of the actual number of refugees. The largest concentration was in the Peshawar region and the largest camps were in the Northwest Frontier Province, now called Khyber Pakhtunkhwa.

There were three hospitals caring for refugees in Peshawar. Mirza was able to find work in one of them, a hospital donated by the European Community. It had a surgery department and a pediatric department. "They had teaching programs for doctors and nurses," Mirza said. "We did general; ear, nose, and throat; and orthopedic surgeries. We operated on about 150 to 200 patients each month."

In addition to treating orthopedic problems caused by trauma, many of Mirza's patients had complications from polio. Due to their living conditions, Afghan refugees represented a high-risk group. "They needed various kinds of surgeries to correct their problems. I was the only orthopedic surgeon for both adults and children. I got a lot of experience."

Mirza remained in Peshawar until the Taliban were routed from power by the U.S.-led invasion. Shortly after Karzai's government came into power, Mirza's hospital was closed and he returned to Afghanistan with his family. Because he was a refugee in Peshawar, he had no relationship with the new Afghan government. Former military members were encouraged to work in non-military hospitals. Mirza took a position with the public hospital in Parwan Province.

Although the hospital in Parwan was a public hospital, it had been built by a French non-governmental organization and was operated by them. Mirza set up the surgery department. "They had never seen the kind of surgery we were able to do."

He remained in Parwan until 2005. One day, one of the hospital's French directors told him about a hospital being built in Kabul by another French organization. This turned out to be the *Mother and Child Hospital* being built by La Chaîne. Mirza initially worked at the hospital as a volunteer, but he was soon selected to be the first orthopedic surgeon. La Chaîne arranged for him to get three months of training at a university pediatric hospital in Paris. When he returned from France, he passed Afghanistan exams to become a trainer in orthopedic surgery. In January 2006, he started work at what had then become known as FMIC.

Mirza's department's accomplishments have steadily increased and his staff has grown to seven, including a second attending orthopedic surgeon. Except for Mirza's brief training in France, all of his team's professional development has been accomplished by visiting mission teams led by orthopedic surgeons from French academic centers. Members of the team began by performing simple consultations and orthopedic procedures, with instruments donated from hospitals in France. Within a few months, they were able to perform surgery to repair fractures, dislocations, and congenital malformations. They had established a reliable orthopedic instrument supply system by 2007 and were able to perform complicated pediatric orthopedic procedures, like the one to straighten Tehmina's spine.

"Spine surgery is one of the big challenges in pediatric orthopedic surgery in Afghanistan," Mirza said. "The majority of pediatric spine pathologies go without treatment and the children eventually get major neurologic and respiratory complications." To address delayed treatment for spinal malformation and deformities, Mirza started a screening system in schools to enable early diagnosis and treatment, possibly avoiding surgery.

Another unique procedure done by Mirza's department is surgical correction of developmental dysplasia, or dislocation, of the hip. This is an abnormal formation of the hip joint, in which the ball on top of the thighbone – the femur – is not held firmly in the socket. According to the American Academy of Orthopedic Surgeons, "The degree of hip looseness, or instability, varies ... In some children, the thighbone is simply loose in the socket at birth. In other children, the bone is completely out of the socket. In still others the looseness worsens as the child grows and becomes more active. While this is usually a birth defect, in Afghanistan it is often the result of a cultural practice of tightly wrapping newborn infants, holding the hips in an abnormal position.

Identification of the condition is often delayed due to the absence of neonatal screening. As a result, children often remain undiagnosed until they begin to walk. At that stage surgical correction is more complicated. Mirza, like his medical colleagues in other FMIC departments, tries to improve early detection of preventable or correctable problems in children by conducting continuing medical education sessions and telemedicine consultations for physicians in other practice settings.

Mirza stresses that the quality of care at FMIC is high because years of effort have gone into training the doctors, nurses, surgeons, and technicians who practice and work there. "The intensive care unit, with its good patient management, oxygen and suction systems, and excellent equipment, is extremely important. The same is true for the operating room. Too many other hospitals just create a room and put some tables, machines, and anesthesia equipment in it," he said. "At FMIC we follow safety and quality rules stringently. We also maintain our equipment. If you buy good equipment and don't operate it properly, or maintain it, it will break down. We have biomedical engineers who maintain the equipment and we train our staff properly on its use. This is what differentiates FMIC."

FRISHTA, SALMA, DR. NAJEEB AND DR. RAHIMA

All of FMIC's services are unique and extraordinary in Afghanistan but, from the beginning, cardiac surgery was the hospital's preeminent service. Eric Cheysson credits La Chaîne's inspiration for that: "It was partly because of Alain Deloche's interests, but we also know that in developing countries it is difficult for them to do this kind of surgery. They can figure out how to do orthopedic surgery, or spine surgery, but what they cannot do is cardiac surgery. In many countries people are dying of untreated cardiac disease. That was the case in Afghanistan."

On June 15, 2011, just over three years from its inauguration, the 1,000th cardiac surgery case was performed at FMIC. From April 2006 through December 2013, a total of 1,683 cardiac surgeries were done. Of those, 876 were open-heart procedures and 807 were closed-heart. Until January 2010, the majority were performed by French mission teams. Since then, the significant majority have been done by an all-Afghan team led by Dr. Najeebullah Bina. Najeeb is an Afghan cardiac surgeon who was trained and lived in France. After participating in several French missions to FMIC, he returned to Afghanistan to join the staff full-time and lead the cardiac surgery program.

Doing pediatric cardiac surgery is complex anywhere. It's even more so in Afghanistan. As is the case with other medical and surgical areas, complications due to the long delay in getting treatment are a major issue. Najeeb describes what he calls the *Afghanistan Syndrome.* "It results from several factors including poverty, geographic isolation, and culture." Najeeb elaborates on the cultural factor. "When a child is first sick, the family starts by taking advice from grandma. This goes on for about a month. Then they go to the Mullah or Imam in their village. From there they go to local private providers in their villages, called basic health workers. Those guys call themselves doctors, but they're not. After about a year, they may decide to seek care in the nearby big city. Eventually, if they are lucky, they will get to FMIC. By then, they are very ill and have serious complications. At best this can result in a delay of months. That's bad enough, but at worst, the delay in getting treatment can be years. Then complications are major."

In the United States, the mortality rate related to cardiac surgery is around 4%. At FMIC it is 3.5%. That is remarkable considering how late children are presented to surgeons at FMIC, and the risk factors associated with them. Some children's conditions are so severe they would be considered too high a risk to even be operated on in Western, developed countries. In Afghanistan, at least at this time in its history, there is no other option than FMIC. Not attempting corrective surgery is a sentence to severe disability, or even death.

Frishta

In June 2012, I was in Afghanistan to chair an FMIC board meeting. Prior to the meeting, I travelled to Bamyan to visit the Bamyan Provincial Hospital, a Ministry of Public Health facility managed by Aga Khan Health Services. FMIC has a Memorandum of Agreement with Bamyan Hospital to provide support to it. This was my fourth trip to Bamyan. The first was in March 2006 when I accompanied His Highness the Aga Khan on a visit there. In subsequent years, as linkages strengthened between Bamyan Hospital and FMIC, I returned to plan the integration of the two hospitals.

While I was in Bamyan Province, I wanted to visit the family of Frishta, daughter of Sayed Sarwar. Frishta, a charming four-year-old, was one of Najeeb Bina's recent open-heart surgery patients. He operated on her just one month earlier to correct a ventricular septal defect. She had this condition since her birth.

In order to understand the issues and complications facing Frishta and her family in maintaining their health and, when necessary, accessing sources of care, it is helpful to understand the environment in which they live.

The city of Bamyan is the capital of Bamyan Province. Its population is around 62,000. Bamyan is approximately 150 miles northwest of Kabul. According to a 2008 handbook published by the U.S. Army Combined Arms Center, the province's total population is nearly 400,000. There are about 55,500 households in the province and households, on average, have seven members. Around eighty percent of the population lives in rural districts. The population is mainly Hazara, followed by Tajik, Tatar, and Pashtun. Hazara are primarily of the Shia Muslim faith. Some believe that Hazaras are descended from Genghis Khan's army. The province is considered one of the most progressive for women's rights and, in 2005, Afghanistan's first female governor was appointed there.

I flew from Washington, D.C., to Bamyan, through Dubai and Kabul. There are no commercial flights from Kabul to Bamyan so the final leg of my trip was on a United Nations Humanitarian Air Service flight, operated in Afghanistan by the World Food Program. My long trip had delays and I had gotten hardly any sleep for two days. I was eight-and-a-half time zones away from home and, despite my lack of sleep, I awoke the first night in my Bamyan hotel – the *Silk Road Hotel* – at around 4 a.m. I was tossing and turning when the muezzin's soft and melodic prayer call began. It echoed off the nearby sandstone cliffs, site of the now-demolished great standing Buddhas, and resonated across the valley. It was soothing and serene.

Bamyan sits in the Hindu Kush range of the Koh-i-Baba Mountains. The Hindu Kush extends about 500 miles east from central Afghanistan to the Pamirs in Tajikistan. Bamyan sits in a green high valley (over 8,000 feet), bounded by ochre cliffs. All around the valley, to the north and to the south, tall mountains are capped with snow many months of the year. I haven't travelled extensively elsewhere in Afghanistan, but Bamyan must stand out as one of the country's most beautiful and tranquil areas. Left to itself, Bamyan valley conveys a sense of peace and serenity. Regrettably, the valley has too often not been left to itself.

Alexander the Great briefly occupied the area around 330 B.C., before moving on to other conquests in the Indian subcontinent. Subsequent rulers introduced Buddhism to the region and it became one of the world's important Buddhist pilgrimage sites. Around the 4th or 5th century A.D., two of the world's largest standing Buddhas were carved into the mountains. Countless caves carved into cliffs facing Bamyan city housed monks and provided shelter for religious pilgrims. In the 18th century, religious zealot soldiers of Aurangzeb, the last great Mughal emperor, defaced the faces of the giant standing Buddhas, but they remained intact and continued to stand as silent sentinels overlooking the valley. More recently, the Buddhas were included in the United Nations Educational, Scientific and Cultural Organization's listing of World Heritage Sites.

The Taliban decided the nearly 1,700 year old statues were idolatrous and, despite pleas from leaders around the civilized world, in March 2001 they methodically and meticulously undertook to destroy them. They destroyed as much as they could with anti-aircraft weapons and tank fire, and finished the job by drilling holes in the statues' torsos and blowing them up. The Taliban's Foreign Minister at the time, Wakil Ahmed Muttawakil, is reported to have said the Taliban had no intention to disrespect any other religion. "We do admit the relics were the cultural heritage of Afghanistan, but the part that contradicts our Islamic beliefs we would not like to have them anymore."

Nothing remains of the great statues now but two ominous mummy-shaped cavities in the hillside. Sometimes, when the sun has a particular slant, the shadows cast inside the cavities create the eerie impression that the Buddhas are still there.

Gull Hussain Baizada is the deputy director of the Rah-e-Abrisham Tourist and Travel Agency in Bamyan. Surprisingly, the purpose of his agency isn't to help people from Bamyan travel abroad. It's to promote tourism in the province. In the 1960s and 1970s, Bamyan was Afghanistan's biggest tourist destination, not only for Afghans but for people from all around the world. According to Gull Hussain, more than 100 automobiles each day arrived with tourists -- so many that there was no housing available for them. Tourism in Bamyan continued until the Soviet invasion, which was followed by the Mujahidin civil war, and Taliban rule. Bamyan suffered very much during those periods.

"How much did those periods of conflict directly affect Bamyan?" I asked.

"There was fighting right in the middle of the city," he said. "Everything was destroyed. Whatever you see here today – these are all new buildings. There is nothing left from the past. And someone was killed in every family. There were group killings, not just one or two people. Large numbers of people were killed at a time."

Tourism reemerged after 2001 due to a brief period of good security, but security deteriorated again after 2005; nevertheless, according to Gull Hussain, tourists still come. "There are no commercial flights and tourists are fewer, but despite the risks they still come. Once anyone visits Bamyan they will not forget it. The people here are very kind and hospitable. They are peaceful people."

Tourism aside, life in Bamyan is not fun and games. Using 2007 and 2008 data, the World Food Program compiled quality of life indicators. Some shocking facts emerge. No one in the entire province has access to safe toilet facilities. Less than one-tenth of households use safe drinking water, and nearly one-tenth of households must travel up to an hour to access safe drinking water. Getting around for any purpose is difficult, whether to access drinking water or urgently needed health services. Only one-fifth of the province's roads are able to take car traffic in all seasons and barely over one-third can only take car traffic in some seasons. In nearly one-fifth of the province there are no roads at all. Access to adequate food is a problem. One-quarter of the population is estimated to receive less than the minimum daily caloric intake necessary to maintain good health. In the whole province, more than three-quarters of the population has low dietary diversity and poor, or very poor, food consumption. The majority of communities, nearly ninety percent, do not have a health worker permanently present in their community. Out of 1,839 villages, only twenty have a health center within their boundaries and only twenty-two have a dispensary. Nearly three-quarters of the population has to travel over six miles to get medical attention.

There is potential wealth in Bamyan Province. There are reportedly massive reserves of mineral resources in Afghanistan. The U.S. government has estimated that Afghanistan holds US$1 trillion in untapped minerals. Some of that is in Bamyan. In a November 2011 article, *Bloomberg Businessweek* reported that a group of Indian companies and Canada's Kilo Goldmines Ltd. were awarded the contract to mine the Hajigak iron ore deposit in Bamyan Province. Hajigak is a series of rugged mountain ridges estimated to hold 1.8 billion metric tons of ore.

If the fruits of this plan ever materialize, the citizens of Bamyan might benefit. In the meantime, it's tough to make a living there. Citing 2007/2008 data, a U.S. Government Accountability Office report found that 44-54% of the province's population falls under the poverty line. The poverty line is defined as "the level of per capita consumption at which the members of the household can be expected to meet their basic needs such as food consumption and housing. In monetary value, the poverty line is less than one dollar per day". Bamyan's isn't the worst poverty level in Afghanistan, but of thirty-three provinces included in the report Bamyan was in the lower third. These were the conditions under which Frishta lived – a young girl with a chronic heart defect since her birth.

Frishta and her family live in Koprok, a village about fifty miles west of Bamyan city. It is located inside the breathtakingly beautiful Band-e-Amir Lake National Park. The centerpieces of the park are six spring-fed, crystalline clear lakes nestled in a spectacularly stark mountain landscape.

I was accompanied on the trip by Dr. Mohammad Nazim, the Clinical Manager of Bamyan Provincial Hospital, and Hamayon Rusoli, the hospital's e-Health Coordinator. Hamayon is a native of Bamyan. During the drive, he recounted his personal experiences with the Taliban. They killed about eighty people from his village, including members of his family.

Frishta's father, Sayed Sarwar, and his cousin met us at a small bazaar just inside the park entrance. They rode with us to their village. They had walked two-and-a-half hours to meet us. We would have never found their village without their guidance. It sits in a rustic green valley surrounded by gentle hills. While the village is small, it is fortunate to have a school and a basic health center. Both were recently constructed and are within a short walk from Frishta's home. Her house is constructed of mud, with a straw roof. The structure contains separate rooms housing relatives of Frishta's family and a common kitchen. As we approached the house I noticed a very large dog chained nearby. "To keep away wolves," I was told.

Frishta and her mother, Sediqa, met us at the front door. They were both dressed in fine and colorful clothes for the occasion of my visit. Frishta has four sisters. The oldest is sixteen years old and married. She lives with her husband. The others – ages fourteen, twelve, and ten – all live at home with Frishta and her parents. The entire family lives, eats, sleeps, and entertains guests in a single room. The room contained no furniture. Large pillows lined the walls and colorful carpets covered the floors. Brightly colored textile objects adorned the walls. A single stove sat at the end of the room near the doorway. The exterior wall had a large opening to the outside. Our meal was passed through that opening after being prepared in the communal kitchen.

Sayed Sarwar welcomed us. My companions from Bamyan Hospital translated our conversation. "Thank you for allowing me to come into your home and talking with me about Frishta's care at FMIC," I told him.

"We are honored to welcome you as our guest," he said. "FMIC takes care of poor people in Afghanistan. We are thankful for FMIC and we are happy you are here."

Frishta's mother remained in the room during the early part of our conversation but she left to join other women in the family to prepare a meal for us. She occasionally returned and joined in the conversation. Frishta stayed in the room for the entire visit. She fidgeted and displayed the discomfort one would expect of a four-year-old, but overall she was amazingly well behaved.

I asked about life in the village and what kind of work Sayed Sarwar did.

"Our village has community animals," Sayed Sarwar told me. "A few cows and sheep. Our villagers take turns watching over them at a grazing meadow. It's about an hour's walk away."

He told me it was his family's turn to care for the animals just before my visit. They were all at the meadow, living in a tent. Frishta, just forty days post-op from open-heart surgery, was with them. I learned, with some embarrassment, that another village family had relieved them of their duties and they had walked back home just to meet with me.

We discussed Frishta's medical history. "When did your family first realize Frishta needed care?" I asked.

"When she was very small she often got pneumonia," Sayed Sarwar replied. "No matter what we fed her she did not grow normally. She could play but she always had chest problems. Finally, her condition got so bad we took her to the health center in Koprok."

His face became worried, a weary expression that any father might wear when recalling a daughter's illness. "The doctor said Frishta had a cardiac problem. He gave her some drugs and multivitamins. He said she should go to Bamyan Hospital."

"I did not see any vehicles in your village when I arrived," I said. "How did you take her there?"

"There is only one motorcycle and a small truck in our village. We have to walk anyplace we go. We walk to a place on the road. It is very far from here. It takes about four hours. It's shorter in the winter because then we can walk across the frozen lake."

"So did you walk the first time you took Frishta to Bamyan Hospital?" I asked. "Did Frishta have to walk too?"

"Yes, we walked. Her mother was with me. I carried Frishta on my back."

I was speechless. Fortunately for Sayed Sarwar – and for Frishta – when they got to the main road his brother, who is employed elsewhere as a driver, passed by. He picked up the family and took them to Bamyan. If that hadn't happened they would have kept walking to Bamyan, with Frishta on her father's back, for two days.

Frishta was admitted to the Bamyan hospital, but she was not able to be treated there. "We are unable to treat her," the doctors told Sayed Sarwar and Sediqa. "She should go to the place called FMIC in Kabul."

"Someone at the hospital told us FMIC was very expensive," Sayed Sarwar said. "We were told Frishta could not be treated there without money. They said we should go to Ata Turk Hospital instead." Ata Turk Hospital is a Ministry of Public Health pediatric hospital located very near FMIC. Its care is not even closely comparable to FMIC. Nevertheless, the family did not know that and they did go to Ata Turk Hospital.

I was distressed to hear that someone at Bamyan Hospital, a place with which FMIC has a formal relationship, would apparently not know about FMIC's patient welfare program and would be directing patients to public hospitals that couldn't treat them. That had to be corrected.

"So what happened at Ata Turk?" I asked.

"They told us they could not treat Frishta and we should go to FMIC. We were very worried about what to do because we had no money."

Sayed Sarwar and Sediqa decided they had no choice but to go to the place called FMIC. They had come this far, perhaps some way could be found for Frishta to be cared for there.

They arrived at FMIC on the weekend and were asked to come back the following day to see a doctor in the heart service. The next day, they saw Dr. Rahima Stanekzai, the head of cardiology. She ordered ultrasound and echocardiogram studies. After discussing Frishta's case with Najeeb, she told the family to go the hospital's patient welfare office for an evaluation of their ability to pay.

"They asked us if we had money, land, homes, houses, or animals. We said we were very poor. We had nothing – only one cow – and there was no one to help us."

The next day they saw Najeeb. He told them all that was needed in order for Frishta to be treated was to donate blood because she needed blood for her surgery. In Afghanistan there are no reliable blood banks or community sources of blood. FMIC must rely on families to provide blood when it is required. Sayed Sarwar gave a pint of blood. Sediqa was told she was anemic and couldn't donate. They contacted a relative at Kabul University who came with two friends and gave more blood, but still more was needed. Finally, staff in FMIC's laboratory and two nurses in the intensive care unit donated blood and, the next morning, Frishta went to surgery.

Sayed Sarwar vividly remembers events surrounding Frishta's surgery. "The doctors took her from her mother's lap and they went to the operating room. Her mother was crying and we were very worried."

It was late afternoon when Najeeb came from the operating room to talk with them. Sayed Sarwar asked him, "How is the patient by the name of Frishta?" Najeeb said her surgery was finished and she was recovering in the intensive care unit. The family could visit her the next morning.

Sayed Sarwar and Sediqa returned to the waiting area but they continued to worry. That evening, he went to a guard. "I said to him, you have children and you know how a father feels. Please let me go to see my child. The guard told me 'no'. He said it was too late, but some foreigners came and asked about the matter. They said I could go see the patient, so the guard let me go. I had to put on some special clothes."

When Sayed Sarwar saw Frishta, she was still asleep from anesthesia. He was concerned that she wasn't conscious. When he returned to Sediqa, she asked him, "How is the child?" He didn't want to upset her so he told her, "She is laughing and she is taking water." Sediqa felt better, but later she went to see Frishta herself and came back crying. "We have lost my child." Sayed Sarwar told her it was good they saw her. After that they went to the hospital yard and slept on the grass.

Sayed Sarwar could not sleep. Around 2 a.m. he was still worried and decided to try to visit Frishta again. After a long discussion with the guards, he went to the on-duty doctors and got permission to visit her again. Once again he put on "special clothes" and went to the intensive care unit. This time Frishta seemed to be stirring a little.

"I thought if I held her hand and she would hold mine, I would know she was alive." Frishta did respond when he held her hand

and he realized she was alive. "But there were needles in many places on her – her chest, her legs, and her arms. She was getting oxygen. I thought she was very worse. I returned to her mother and she asked, 'How is she now?' I told her, she is laughing now."

Sayed Sarwar and Sediqa went together to see Frishta the next morning. Najeeb was with her and gave them a toy for her, a stuffed bear. After that they knew Frishta was going to be okay.

I was engrossed by Sayed Sarwar's story. There was so much drama in it and so many lessons to be learned, beginning with the saga of simply getting to FMIC. The cultural gap of the family's understanding of the course of Frishta's treatment was revealing and highlighted the importance of ensuring the best communications between doctors and families. I had to follow-up on that. And, finally, Sayed Sarwar's sensitivity about Sediqa's anxieties was tender and touching.

Sayed Sarwar reflected on the miracle of Frishta's care at FMIC. "When she was sick, her mother and I used to wonder what would happen to her when we were gone but now we don't worry about that. Now we can hope for a better life for her."

My traveling companions and I arrived at Frishta's home at about noon. I knew we would be served the finest meal the family could provide us. I also knew it would be beyond their means, but Afghan custom demanded they offer us the best they possibly could and that I graciously accept it. As our conversation wound down, Frishta's mother began supervising delivery of the meal to us through the opening in the exterior wall. It was sumptuous. We were served juice and soup for a starter, followed by mutton, yogurt, yogurt cheese, cucumbers, tomatoes, and onions. No utensils other than a soup spoon were used for eating. Everything was scooped up with naan, the delicious Afghan flat bread. My colleagues from Bamyan Hospital had no reservations about diving into the meal with gusto. Dessert was a delicious, juicy watermelon. Watermelons were in season. I had seen them stacked for sale at every corner market, and they were served at nearly every meal.

I don't normally eat a big mid-day meal. I ate as much as I could, but I don't think I came close to eating as much as was expected of me. I knew the effort and expense that had gone into the meal, and I hoped I hadn't offended the family's hospitality.

After lunch, I asked permission to take some pictures of Frishta. Sayed Sarwar agreed and was pleased to join in them. He asked me, however, to not take pictures of Sediqa. In Kabul, I am sometimes permitted to take pictures of female family members, but that is not common in rural areas. It's not even common for female members to meet with strangers, so I was privileged that Sediqa met me.

Frishta's circumstances represent two common obstacles to providing good health care in Afghanistan: poverty and geographic isolation in harsh and remote settings. Often there are not good roads. Sometimes there are no roads at all. Even if there are, most people don't have vehicles. For many families there is no recourse other than to walk long distances through mountainous terrain. It's the way their life has always been and they have no reason to think it will change. On rare occasions when public transportation is available, it is too expensive for poor families to afford. A bus trip from Bamyan to Kabul costs 4,000 Afghanis (AFN), or about US$80.00. Modest hotel accommodation in Kabul costs about 77 AFN a night – around US$1.50. These are miniscule amounts by some standards but, when you are poor and have just one cow, it's a fortune.

Bamyan Hospital paid for the family's first transportation to Kabul, but the family paid for their own hotel. Just before my visit they had returned to Kabul for a follow-up appointment. That time, they stayed for several days at Kate's Kids' House at no cost to them. After Frishta's examination, they were asked to return again in another month.

"What should I do now?" he asked almost pleadingly. "I have already lost all I have for Frishta! I have no money to make another trip."

I told Dr. Nazim I would leave money on deposit at Bamyan Hospital to pay the travel costs of Frishta's next visit to FMIC. I thought that was an appropriate "visit gift" to compensate the family for all the disruption they had suffered to meet with me, and the cost they incurred to provide such a lavish meal. Dr. Nazim and I agreed that he would personally coordinate their next visit to FMIC and he would ensure space was available for them at The Kids' House. All the family's costs for treatment and lodging would be covered.

Dr. Nazim and I discussed the possibility of expanding the use of Bamyan Hospital's telemedicine linkage with FMIC so that patients like Frishta wouldn't even have to make follow-up visits to FMIC. Bamyan Hospital and its patients had already benefited greatly from the linkage, but there was still greater potential to reduce the need for travel between the locations. It would require doctors at the two sites to agree on cardiac surgery follow-up protocols. Bamyan doctors could conduct lab or x-ray tests required by the FMIC specialists and the "visits" could be conducted via the telemedicine linkage. Some follow-up care would require that patients be physically present at FMIC, but if even some of the necessity for travel could be eliminated, that would be a major breakthrough. In order for the e-Health system to work best, some investment would be needed to train doctors and other health professionals at Bamyan, or to purchase required equipment that was presently not available there. Those investments should be justified by the reduction in costs families would incur or, importantly, by reducing morbidity or mortality incurred by poor patients failing to get the required follow-up care. I was excited about the opportunity to pursue these initiatives with management of the two hospitals.

My visit ended by walking with the family from their house to the village's Basic Health Center. Dr. Nazim wanted to personally examine Frishta's chest and listen to her heart. His examination revealed that everything was good. That was a satisfying end to the visit.

While I stood waiting in the corridor outside the health center examining room, I was confronted with another unfortunate reality facing Afghanistan's children. Several youngsters, all around four to six years old, were waiting to see the clinic's sole doctor. It was obvious they had assorted chronic illnesses and serious disabilities. They were dirty and their skin was crusted with grime and inflammation. Some were crippled. They shuffled in and waited stoically and silently. It was possible their fathers had brought them to the clinic because the word was out in the village that a foreigner was there. The chances were slim that anything would be done, ever, to relieve them of their suffering. I could see in their eyes that they knew that. Their ailments and conditions were not new. They looked at me warily. I was somebody new. Maybe I would help them. Tragically that wasn't going to happen. I couldn't help them. Nothing was going to alleviate their suffering. Everything was stacked against them. Some would die before they reached adolescence. Others would carry their burdens for their entire lives. The resignation I saw in their eyes caused tightness in my chest and the lump that formed in my throat made it hard to swallow. It didn't seem right that any of God's children should suffer so much.

When I returned to Kabul I discussed Frishta's case with Najeeb. Tests that he and Dr. Rahima performed when she arrived at FMIC had led them to conclude she had suffered since birth with a ventricular septal defect, VSD, commonly known as a hole in the heart. Najeeb thinks Frishta's condition was caused by her mother's advanced age, about thirty-seven, and poor nutrition during her pregnancy. Sometimes the condition self-corrects as the child grows older. If it doesn't, open-heart surgery is often indicated. If VSD is not detected and corrected early in life it can lead to severe complications, even death. Frishta had developed the complication pulmonary hypertension, high blood pressure in the arteries of the lungs. Najeeb believes that without treatment she would have become increasingly ill and would not have survived beyond fifteen or sixteen years.

Frishta's surgery involved opening her chest and closing the hole in her heart with a patch. The defect was corrected and closed carefully under microsurgery procedures. Najeeb remembers the problem Frishta's family had in providing blood for her surgery.

"Do you remember that FMIC staff donated blood for her?" I asked.

"Of course I do," he said. "It is not unusual for FMIC staff to contribute blood for cardiac surgery patients. Cardiac surgery is not just a profession in Afghanistan. At FMIC it is something filled with emotion and feelings. When we need blood, the call goes through all of FMIC's departments – to the guards, the cooks, housekeepers, and nurses. Everybody in the hospital knows that a cardiac patient needs blood. ICU nurses and people from the lab provided blood for Frishta. It is a kind of solidarity and friendship within FMIC. It is unbelievable."

Najeeb is confident that because of Frishta's surgery she will have a normal life. He fixed her heart but she won his. "From the day she arrived, until she left, she was always smiling. She won lots of hearts."

Frishta was in the hospital for seven days. The total cost of her surgery was approximately US$4,180.00. The cost of her procedure in the U.S. would be approximately US$50,000.00. Her family had no capacity to pay. Eighty percent of the cost of her care was paid for by funds contributed by La Chaîne through Kate's project, and twenty percent was paid through the FMIC's patient welfare program.

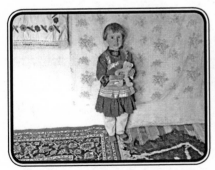
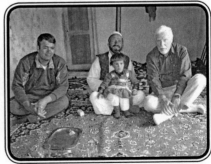

Frishta with Teddy Bear from FMIC   *Lee with Frishta, her father, and uncle*

Salma

After the board meeting in Kabul, I flew to Badakhshan Province, again on a UN humanitarian service aircraft. In Badakhshan, I wanted to visit the Faizabad Provincial Hospital, another hospital managed by Aga Khan Health Services and supported by FMIC. I also wanted to visit the family of a young cardiac patient from Badakhshan: Salma, daughter of Habibullah. Salma had surgery at FMIC in December 2010 to correct a congenital heart condition.

Badakhshan's capital city, Faizabad, has a population of about 50,000. Faizabad is located approximately 195 miles from Kabul. The Kokcha River divides the so-called new area of the city from what the locals call "Old Faizabad". Badakhshan Province is nestled in the Hindu Kush and Pamir Mountain ranges. The mountains surrounding Faizabad are among the tallest in the world. Seven of Afghanistan's ten highest mountains, including its highest, are in Badakhshan. All are around 20,000 feet in height. The winter of 2011-2012 had seen heavy snowfalls and, when we arrived in July, the peaks were still capped with snow and the Kokcha River was fast-flowing from the melt-off.

Badakhshan is an oddly-shaped province located in the northeastern region of Afghanistan. It shares international borders with Tajikistan, Pakistan, and China. My Rorschach ink-blot interpretation of the province's silhouette sees a mythical condor rising up in flight out of Afghanistan. The condor's long neck stretches far to the east and it has captured a small chunk of the western edge of China in its mouth. Badakhshan's unique shape is no accident, nor is it dictated by geography. It is a purely political contrivance. In the late nineteenth century, Britain was concerned that Russia would encroach into its colonial crown jewel, India, from

Central Asia. To preclude this, Britain sought to create a buffer zone, known today as the *Wakhan Corridor*, between Russian-controlled territory and India. The connived borders separated large populations with common tribal, ethnic, and religious characteristics. One population affected was the Ismailis. The Wakhan Corridor drove a wedge between Ismailis in Afghanistan, Tajikistan, and what is now Northern Pakistan.

Estimates of Badakhshan's population vary widely, but most place it near 900,000. Nearly ninety-six percent of the population lives in rural districts. The Ministry of Rural Rehabilitation and Development's 2007 *Provincial Profile* estimated there were 134,137 households in the province, and that those households, on average, had six members. The majority population is Tajik, with Uzbek and Kyrgyz minorities. The majority religion is Sunni Muslim.

In some ways, the quality of life for Salma in Badakhshan is slightly better than for Frishta in Bamyan but, in other ways, it is worse. It is estimated that, on average, only thirteen percent of households use safe drinking water. One in six households must travel up to an hour to access drinking water, and twelve percent of households travel up to six hours to get drinking water. Only one percent of the households in Badakhshan have access to electricity. Transportation is poor to non-existent, and getting around the province for any reason is difficult. Barely one-quarter of roads in the province are able to handle car traffic in all seasons and in just over half of the province there are no roads at all. This is even worse than in Bamyan where only twenty percent of the province has no roads.

Badakhshan was one of only two Afghan provinces never occupied by the Taliban. As a result, many of its educational institutions remained intact. This good fortune left it with one of the highest literacy rates in Afghanistan – thirty-one percent. While that number is low, Afghanistan's overall literacy rate is barely over twenty-eight percent. The Badakhshan *Provincial Profile* reported there were 430 primary and secondary schools in the province catering for 216,000 students. Boys account for fifty-four percent of the students, and ninety-two percent of the schools are boys' schools. As elsewhere in Afghanistan, Badakhshan men have the advantage over women. Nearly two in five men are literate compared to one in five women.

Badakhshan's main commercial activity is trade in agricultural and livestock products. There are many fertile valleys in which crops are grown. Despite that, around two people in five receive less than the minimum daily caloric intake necessary to maintain good health. Around three-quarters of the population has low dietary diversity and poor, or very poor, food consumption. These numbers are worse than Bamyan's.

The 2008 U.S. Army Combined Arms Center handbook reported that Badakhshan had forty-eight health centers and two hospitals with 191 beds. Data that same year showed that seventy-five Ministry of Public Health doctors and 339 other public sector health professionals were working in the province. Nevertheless, the majority of communities do not have a health worker permanently present. Sixteen percent of the population must travel more than three miles to reach the nearest health facility. Sick or well, much of that travel is done by walking or riding a donkey over arduous mountain terrain in all seasons.

Badakhshan's poverty level is among the worst in Afghanistan, which makes it among the worst in the world. The U.S.

Government Accounting Office (GAO) report on poverty and major crop production pegs over one-half to three-quarters (55-76%) of Badakhshan's population as living below the poverty line. This places it in the lower one-fifth of Afghanistan's thirty-three provinces.

Through all of Afghanistan's recent conflicts, Badakhshan Province has been a relatively peaceful and secure place, at least compared to the rest of the country. The conditions "peaceful" and "secure" are relative terms in Afghanistan. On August 7, 2010, eight foreigners and two Afghans were found shot dead in Badakhshan. Six Americans, one Briton, and a German were among the foreigners. All had worked for the International Assistance Mission (IAM), a charity providing eye care throughout Afghanistan. An IAM spokesman said the group had been conducting eye clinics for two-and-a-half weeks in the neighboring province of Nuristan, at the invitation of communities there. They were returning to Kabul via Badakhshan because they thought that would be their safest route.

The tragic event struck close to home for those of us involved with FMIC. IAM had founded and operated the forty-bed NOOR Eye Hospital, abutting FMIC on the Kabul Medical University campus. The facility was excellent and, like FMIC, provided high quality care of an international standard. I had visited that facility and met the highly professional and dedicated members of the NOOR team, some of whom were killed in the attack in Badakhshan.

The morning after I arrived in Faizabad, I departed for the village of Nawa, in the Jurm district. That's where Salma, FMIC's young cardiac surgery patient, lived. In December 2010, Salma had a closed-heart procedure to prepare her for eventual open-heart surgery to correct a congenital condition known as Tetralogy of Fallot.

I was accompanied on the drive to Nawa by the clinical director at Faizabad Hospital. He would translate for me during the conversation with Salma and her family. Dr. Abdi is from Badakhshan and is an Ismaili. He said the trip to Nawa Village would take three to four hours and would be "very difficult." We would often be in a valley alongside the river and "between two big mountains." It sounded fabulous.

During the first few minutes of the trip, we wound through "New" Faizabad on well-paved streets. We crossed a bridge over the rapidly coursing and muddy Kokcha River into "Old" Faizabad, where the streets were less well-paved but still comfortable to ride on. Within minutes, we came to the edge of town – and the end of paved roads. For most of the rest of the day, we rode on gravel and dirt roads alongside the Kokcha River. Sometimes we were in it. As mentioned previously, the winter of 2011-2012 had been exceptionally harsh with much snowfall. In July, the snow was still melting and the river was turbulent and sometimes overflowed its banks. At one point it washed over our road. Thanks to our four-wheel drive vehicle we were able to cross through water above our vehicle's wheels.

Several road construction projects had been completed or were underway in Badakhshan. In 2010, the U.S. Agency for International Development (USAID) completed a sixty-four mile long road connecting Badakhshan's Kesham district with Faizabad. Several other projects were underway. The new roads would aid the local economy and quality of life by reducing the costs of travel, as well as the travel time. Goods and products would be more efficiently transported to markets and, hopefully, individuals would have better access to needed health care services.

As we travelled east we stayed close to the Koprok River. At times, we were high on hillsides overlooking wide fertile valleys. We saw ample evidence of Badakhshan's abundant crops. Apples and cherries were in season and wheat and barley were being harvested in fields all along our route.

We arrived at Nawa Village just before noon. Our arrival was anticipated. Salma's father, Habibullah, was waiting for me alongside the road in what seemed to be the center of the village. Our short walk to Salma's house followed a bucolic, shaded path bordered on one side by a mud and stone wall, and on the other by small trees and a bubbling stream. At the end of the path, I was led through a portal in the wall and entered a small residential compound. Habibullah invited me into a room where Salma and a male relative stood waiting. Salma's mother was not present. During the few hours I spent in their home, talking and having tea with Salma, her father, and other male family members, Salma's mother, Simin, never made an appearance.

Salma was dressed in a floral-designed salwar kameez with a long green scarf covering her head. She had large brown eyes which, in the beginning of my visit, she frequently averted. The longer we were together, the more she ventured to make direct eye contact with me. She was appropriately modest, even shy, but she didn't appear unnerved by being the center of attention.

The room we were in had no furniture. A deep red carpet covered the floor and cushions lined the walls. A few decorative fabrics adorned the walls. Habibullah said their home had two other small rooms, a kitchen and one small toilet room. He invited me to sit on cushions stacked along one wall. He and Salma settled onto cushions across from me. Tea was brought in on a tray and we began our conversation.

I had brought a box of chocolate candy for the family, which I handed to Habibullah. "You are very kind to invite me to your home," I said. "I look forward to discussing Salma's illness and her care at FMIC with you."

"Thank you," he said, accepting my gift with a beaming look of surprise. "You are welcome in our home. You have come far to talk with us about Salma."

I asked Habibullah if Salma had brothers and sisters.

"Yes," he replied as he poured tea into a small cup and handed it to me. "She is one of eight children in our family. The oldest is fifteen years and the youngest fifteen days." Wow! I thought that was likely one of the reasons why Simin didn't join us.

"Can you tell me what Salma's life was like before she had her surgery?" I asked.

Habibullah's manner grew serious and he shook his head, as if remembering something he would just as soon forget. "It was terrible," he said. "She had been ill all her life. From her birth she was very small and her color was almost totally black."

Her color would have been due to poor circulation and lack of oxygen. After sipping my tea I asked, "Had you ever tried to get care for her before she came to FMIC?"

"Oh yes, we took her to a doctor and he told us she had a heart problem. He gave us some medicine and said she should use it. We used it for two or three years but then stopped. We had to buy the medicine and, after three years, we had no money to keep buying it."

I wondered what kind of medicine had been prescribed for Salma. Apparently it hadn't done her much good. For the next several years she received no treatment.

"Salma's condition during all of that time sounds like it must have been difficult for her," I said. "What was it like for your family?"

"It was bad," he said. "From the time she was three until she was eleven, she could not walk. She had no strength or energy. Her mother carried her everywhere she went. She could not go to school. She had no life at all."

I looked at Salma. Her color was obviously much better, but it still didn't look to me like it was up to one hundred percent. She briefly glanced at me, but then averted her eyes downward. Habibullah was speaking in Dari and his comments were being translated for me. She would have been following our conversation.

"How did you find out about FMIC, and what led you to seek care there?" I asked.

"When Salma was eleven years old, we found out about FMIC from a relative who works there," Habibullah said. "He told us it would be possible for her to get an operation that might make her well."

Habibullah gathered together what money he could and went

to Kabul. "We went from Jurm to Faizabad by a small car. From there we took a big bus to Kabul. Salma sat in the back of the bus." I tried to picture Salma – unable to walk by herself and nearly black in color – making that kind of trip.

At FMIC they were seen by the cardiologist, Dr. Rahima. She conducted tests and knew cardiac surgery would be required. Unfortunately, even though the family had a relative who worked at FMIC, they had not made advance arrangements before just showing up. Dr. Rahima told them none of the cardiac surgeons were in Kabul and the operation could not be scheduled at that time. She said they should return to Badakhshan and they would be notified when it could be performed. They returned to Badakhshan and waited. Finally they were contacted to return to see Najeeb Bina.

Habibullah didn't have money to make the return trip. He went to a local microfinance office in Badakhshan and borrowed 50,000 AFN – about US$1,000. He used some of this money to take Salma back to Kabul.

I said I thought microfinance loans were to be strictly used for business investment purposes. Habibullah acknowledged this was true. "This money is supposed to be only for business, for working, but when I took it, it was not for business. A woman in the office saw our dire situation and talked to the manager," he said. "He agreed to give us the money. I still haven't paid all of it back. Almost 30,000 AFN still has to be repaid."

When the family returned to FMIC, Salma was seen by Najeeb and Dr. Rahima. "They told us Salma needed a diagnostic test that could not be done at FMIC, a catheterization of her heart.

We had to go to Peshawar for that. That cost another 30,000 AFN. I got this money from some Badakhshani people who were living in Pakistan. They helped us with this."

This extra travel by a poor family with a very sick child was definitely not good. Unfortunately, FMIC did not have a cardiac catheterization unit. If that level of diagnosis was needed, the closest facility was in Peshawar. Finally, with the exam results from Peshawar, Najeeb decided he could perform Salma's surgery.

"How did it go?" I asked. "How was her recovery?"

"She had internal bleeding for one or two days, but Dr. Bina immediately put a tube in. When she got better, he saw she was not walking. She just stayed in bed. I told him she had not walked in nearly nine years. He said please start her walking."

I expressed my empathy with Salma. "She had barely been able to walk for most of her life and it must have been daunting to get up and be active right after heart surgery."

Habibullah smiled. "Well she did it." At FMIC there is a ramp going from x-ray up to the wards. In one day she went up and down the ramp many times!"

I wondered what the family's life was like after Salma came home. "Was she able to lead a more normal life?" I asked.

Habibullah was delighted with the changes that occurred in the family's and Salma's lives after her surgery. "Before the operation she could not go to the bazaar, to school, or even to other houses," he said. "All the family had to take care of her all the time. Now she can walk and she goes to school nearly every day. Only on some days she doesn't go when the weather is very hot. She has friends. Other children from the neighborhood go with her. She is very happy."

I looked at Salma, but saw no visible expression of her alleged happiness. She looked directly at me and seemed to be studying me, wondering what I might be thinking about all her father was telling me. I smiled and nodded approvingly at her. Without changing her expression she looked away.

Starting life anew hadn't been easy for her. She had missed so much school that she had to start in early grades with small children. Since her surgery she had attended school for nearly two years and was in the second grade. Habibullah urged the teacher to move her into a higher grade.

"The teacher says she is very intelligent. I asked her to move Salma into a class with older children. She is not happy to be in class with the very small, small children. Salma likes school and she wants to continue her studies. She likes to study the Persian language."

Despite her improved condition after her first surgery, Salma's treatment was not complete. She required a second procedure. Habibullah was not sure how this could happen.

"They told us her operation should be done in two phases. She should have had the second operation after one year, but again I have no money. I am not able to take her back to FMIC. We cannot go to private doctors either. I was in a pharmacy in the bazaar. I only got one tablet for her. The pharmacist asked why I didn't get one packet. I said I can only afford one tablet."

I told Habibullah it was critical that Salma have her second operation as soon as possible. "She should have already had it by now,"
I stressed. "It is very important. Because of your family's low income, I am sure her next surgery and care at FMIC would be paid
for almost entirely by the patient welfare program. Arrangements
could be made for you to stay at The Kids' House at no cost."

I asked Dr. Abdi what the cost of transportation from Nawa
Village to Kabul and back would be. He said it would cost about
US$90.00. I told Habibullah I would deposit that amount, in
Salma's name, at Faizabad Provincial Hospital to cover their trans-
portation. No further cost should be incurred.

Dr. Abdi said he would work with Habibullah and FMIC to
schedule Salma's return visit. Habibullah said he was very happy I
came. "Inshallah we will get her second operation."

I noted that Habibullah has a large family, debts, and uncertain
income. I asked how he is able to provide for his family under these
circumstances. How does he earn his living? What is his business?

Habibullah said he is blessed to own his house and he has a small
woodworking shop in the local bazaar. He buys unfinished products
from another shop and finishes them to re-sell in his shop. He has
owned his business for six years. Now he says that is all going to end.

"The government is going to build a road right through where
my shop is located. I will soon have no business. I am trying to
find some other work to do."

With another serving of tea, and some delicious locally grown
cherries and nuts, our discussion turned to war and politics.

Salma's family and most of the residents in the region are Tajik Sunnis. "There is a village not too far from here where Ismailis live, maybe about fifteen to twenty families. All the rest are Sunni."

I asked whether the village was affected by war during the recent decades. "The Russians had one of their big bases in Faizabad but they never came to our district and Nawa Village," he answered. During the civil war the area changed hands several times, but there was only limited fighting among the Mujahidin. Limited as the fighting was, Habibullah's brother was killed in it.

Habibullah's face had a proud and defiant look when he said the Taliban never occupied Badakhshan Province. "It was the only province Taliban never got into. Massoud was the defender of this area."

Habibullah is concerned about what will happen after 2014, when the international military forces leave. He is afraid the government cannot control the situation and there is no Massoud here now to defend the area. "Maybe again there will be war. The people here cannot live with the Taliban. Taliban are not of our people."

Before we departed, I took pictures of Salma and her father. I thanked Habibullah for his family's hospitality and said I looked forward to hearing about Salma's successful second surgery.

My next trip to Kabul was four months later. When I arrived at FMIC, I was informed that Salma was in the hospital and had her follow-up surgery just a day before I arrived. I was delighted to know they had returned for her second surgery and anxious to know how it went. I immediately checked on her status and found she was recovering in the intensive care unit.

When I walked into the intensive care unit, Salma was sitting up in bed and her mother was helping her sip water. Salma looked great. In Badakhshan I was concerned that her cheeks seemed excessively flushed. Now, just one day after surgery, she was bright-eyed and alert and her complexion looked normal. She was pleased to see me and was more willing to talk with me than when I visited her at her home. I was amazed about her apparent good condition so soon after open-heart surgery.

Although I had not met Salma's mother, Simin, during my visit at Nawa, at FMIC she was very happy to meet me and had no reservations about talking with me. One of the intensive care unit nurses translated for us. Simin said she was happy the family was able to return for Salma's second surgery and she was relieved her daughter was doing so well.

Later in the day, I talked with Najeeb. He was pleased with Salma's post-operative status, but said her case turned out to be more unique and complicated than he expected it would be. He explained that when he saw Salma in 2010 she was in a very severe cyanotic state. "She was not able to walk on her own for even a few meters and she was weaker than other kids of her age."

Based on their diagnostic work-up, he and Dr. Rahima determined Salma had Tetralogy of Fallot (TOF), a common congenital cyanotic heart defect and the most common cause of blue baby syndrome. In western countries, children with TOF typically have open-heart surgery performed in their infancy or early childhood. Untreated TOF is commonly fatal before age twenty but, with early open-heart surgery, patients have an excellent chance of survival.

When Najeeb first saw Salma, he considered whether he would do a total correction of her problem in a single operation or do it in two stages. If he did the procedure in two stages the first one would involve inserting a special kind of shunt to correct the pulmonary stenosis. Inserting the shunt is a closed-heart, palliative procedure. It involves putting a special prosthesis between the subclavian and pulmonary arteries to enable improved blood flow to the lungs. That improves the patient's oxygen levels, and the increased flow improves the vasculature in the lungs. If he went this route, a permanent repair would have to be done at a later date, usually within a year.

"So what influenced you to make the choice you did in Salma's case?" I asked.

"In the West," Najeeb explained, "this kind of choice-making doesn't often happen, because patients there haven't gone so long without treatment and secondary complications and conditions haven't had time to develop. You would never find a ten- or eleven-year-old patient with TOF. That would be extraordinary. Surgeons in the West follow the *Rule of 3*: the patient should be three kilograms, three months, and the diameter of the pulmonary artery should be three millimeters. When those criteria are met surgeons will do the surgery. It is a different situation in Afghanistan."

Najeeb said his waiting list for heart surgery had kids on it that are nearly adults. He has different strategies for young children than for older ones. "I will immediately do total correction on small kids because the pulmonary arteries are still well-developed. They have good anatomy and clinical fitness. For older children, I prefer they stay alive with a shunt and return for a second surgery, rather than taking a big risk that may cause complications we cannot treat."

Najeeb decided to take a conservative approach with Salma and do the shunt first. "When I see such severe stenosis I will do the surgery in two stages. Life for my patients is all about flow. With the blockage the small branches inside the lungs do not develop. They stay under-developed. The shunt provides oxygen and it expands and develops the pulmonary arteries." He anticipated that Salma's second surgery would involve removing the shunt and repairing the hole in her heart by putting a patch over it. Under the best of circumstances, this would be complicated enough for a patient at such an advanced age and with so much progression of problems.

When Najeeb opened Salma's chest and closely examined her, he found the problem was much more complicated. Her heart had coped with her condition for so many years that the extent of the defects was magnified. The pulmonary stenosis, or blockage, was severe. Because the right ventricle had to work so hard and for so long to push blood through the stenosis, it had developed an extraordinarily large mass of hypertrophied (excess) muscle and the actual ventricle was very small, or compressed. The left ventricle was, in his words, "huge." To complicate things further, the hole in her heart was anything but small. It was large and uniquely shaped. Najeeb called it a "W Committed VSD", meaning the defect spanned both chambers instead of just being confined to the dome of the ventricle.

Najeeb had to accomplish complicated, multi-faceted repairs of several severe conditions. He had to remove the shunt from the first operation and construct a new pulmonary trunk. He had to increase the capacity of the right ventricle, which was diminished from the excessive muscle pushing onto it. This involved completely opening it --"another huge risk," according to Najeeb -- and placing a large pericardial patch on it to increase its size.

"Can you imagine a small pocket? To increase the capacity I open it and put on another patch of tissue so it becomes larger."

Another difficult aspect of the surgery was dealing with the hypertrophic muscle which was blocking the right ventricle's access to the lungs. "You have this enormous bundle of muscle that you have to cut, but at the same time you don't want to cut it because you could reduce the capacity of the right ventricle. The functional unit of the cardiac mechanism is muscle. If you remove muscle it means you are reducing capacity."

Finally, Najeeb had to close a much larger and problematically shaped VSD, which was extending out of both chambers. This involved applying a special "W" shaped patch. "It was a big challenge for us to get the right kind of patch on or otherwise everything would blow out. Fortunately, we were able to diagnose the situation on the table and we had already cut this kind of patch."

Najeeb said Salma's condition is uncommon, occurring in only about one in more than 5,000 cases. Out of more than 1,200 cardiac surgeries done at FMIC, there has been no other case like it. He ranks it as one of the most difficult. He realizes that surgeons in the West may not agree with his criteria and methodology. "I'm sure some will say I am wrong, maybe even mad. They may say I am doing surgery like they did in the 60s and 70s. But we have good results and I think what we do is justified in Afghanistan."

Najeeb did his job well and the outcome was excellent. Salma was already on her way to a good recovery when I saw her just one day after surgery. I couldn't help but be impressed. This was an extraordinary accomplishment for an all-Afghan surgical team working in Kabul.

I visited Salma several times during the next couple of days, and she looked better each time. She was transferred out of the intensive care unit in only three days. Eight days after her admission she was discharged from the hospital. She and her parents would stay at The Kids' House for a few more days, where she would convalesce and return for outpatient visits until she was deemed fit enough to return to her village in Badakhshan.

The total cost of Salma's first operation in 2010 was 120,000 AFN, or about US$2,500.00. Based on FMIC's assessment of the family's ability to pay, the charge was reduced to just one-quarter of that – about US$625.00. Habibullah used some of the microfinance loan for this. The rest was covered by the hospital's welfare program. The total cost of her second surgery was 223,311 AFN – US$ 4,379.00. FMIC's patient welfare program covered that entire amount.

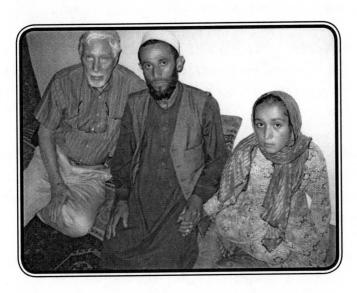

Lee with Salma and her father

Dr. Najeeb

When I talk with the doctors and nurses at FMIC, I am deeply impressed by their patriotism and dedication to their country. They have their personal dreams and aspirations, but nearly all of them also care about and want to contribute to the quality of life of their fellow countrymen. Because of the consequences of their country's long period of war, they fear they may never have the enabling conditions to fulfill their potential. Many see FMIC as a possible catalyst to enable them to do that. Najeeb's story is a case in point.

Najeeb was born in Kandahar. Compared to many Afghans his life was one of privilege. Doors of opportunity were open to him. His father was a physician who rose to be a four-star general in the Afghan military before retiring in January 2011. His mother was a professor of literature at Kabul University. Due to his father's military postings, his family moved frequently around Afghanistan.

Najeeb's fit and trim physique attests to his athletic skill. For over five years he played soccer on the Afghan national team. He had a promising career as a footballer, but he decided instead to study medicine.

I asked him what affect the Soviet invasion had on his family. "Others have told me that life in Afghanistan wasn't really all that bad under the Soviets. What do you think? Was your family's life disrupted?"

"Much of the peace in our life was disturbed," he answered. "My father managed hospitals. During the invasion he was leading military hospitals in Kabul and Jalalabad. Doctors were respected regardless of what side they were on. But the Communists saw my family as aristocrats and we weren't greatly appreciated by them and weren't treated well."

Some members of Najeeb's family were arrested and others just disappeared. His father was transferred to a battalion located near Jalalabad, close to the Pakistan border. In 1983, his father was seriously wounded during an attack on an ambulance in which he was riding. He spent a year in the hospital. He lost one eye and could no longer fully use his left hand. Najeeb thinks Soviets were responsible for the attack on the ambulance.

Najeeb admits that the Soviets maintained much of Afghanistan's social infrastructure and systems during their occupation. "They were here ten or eleven years. During that time they kept things working pretty well. They came and saw a strong government system already in place. They changed it some to fit their own wishes, but it was working, at least for people here in Kabul or in big cities. I am not saying it was a good system but at least there was a system. At least people had enough to eat and clothes to wear."

Najeeb's life became more complicated when the Soviets pulled out. The civil war started soon afterwards, and the Mujahidin came to Kabul in April 1992. He was in his third year attending Kabul Medical University.

"Suddenly people all around us divided into factions," he said. I remember the first day of the university opening. Twenty minutes after it opened, fights broke out on opposite sides of the campus, just one hundred meters from where FMIC is now. We had to run. We couldn't come back to classes for two years. Everything was closed."

During this hiatus in his education, Najeeb's family was living in Kabul where his father was running a military hospital. That enabled Najeeb to continue working in medicine. "I wasn't trained enough to do surgery, but I could work in clinics with physicians and surgeons. My father helped me. He always said, 'Just wait. It will change. We have to accept this.' My father was the best model for me."

After two years, the Kabul Medical University began classes again and Najeeb returned to medical school. Shortly after he returned, the campus was hit by a rocket attack during Mujahidin fighting. Six of his classmates were killed. "At that point I seriously considered whether I wanted to stop my medical education. I thought about leaving medicine and pursuing a career playing soccer. My father said to forget that. There was no future for that in Afghanistan. Maybe there would be in Iran, Turkey, or Dubai, but not Afghanistan. I accepted his guidance to continue my education and stay in medicine."

Najeeb completed his medical education and passed the government entrance examination for thoracic surgery. "I chose that specialty because it was related to the heart. I was especially interested in cardiac surgery. It was my dream to be the one to develop cardiac surgery in Afghanistan."

In 2002, Najeeb was awarded a scholarship at the University of Lyon in France to pursue his doctorate degree in cardiovascular surgery. "The University of Lyon had a long relationship with Afghanistan. It stopped when the Soviets occupied our country. A delegation from Lyon came to Kabul in 2002, to restart the relationship. They went to teaching hospitals all around Kabul looking for young surgeons and physicians. Dr. Rahima Stanekzai and

I were the first doctors selected after ten years. They asked what I wanted to study and I said cardiac surgery. Dr. Rahima went to Paris to study cardiology and I went to Lyon."

From January 2003 until January 2007, Najeeb completed two Masters Degrees and his PhD. In 2007, during a trip back to Kabul to visit his family, he heard about FMIC and learned that the French NGO, La Chaîne de l'Espoir, was involved with it. When he returned to France he contacted the organization. The match seemed perfect. Since 2006, La Chaîne had carried out a pediatric cardiac surgery program in Kabul, but exclusively with French surgeons and mission teams. The opportunity to create a center staffed by Afghans seemed possible. Najeeb's dream might be realized.

In 2008, while still completing his training in France, Najeeb first worked at FMIC as a member of one of La Chaîne's cardiac mission teams. He joined FMIC full time in January 2010. One month later, the first open-heart surgery case was conducted by a team comprised entirely of Afghans.

The Afghan team consists of Najeeb, a perfusionist (Mohammad Din), an anesthetist, two junior doctors, and two nurses. Mohammad Din was trained for six years by perfusionists with French mission teams, and training for him was arranged at the Chennai Cardiac Center in India. Since 2012, he has performed more than 550 open-heart cases under Najeeb's supervision. He is the first Afghan perfusionist ever accredited and certified by the Ministry of Public Health. Dr. Nassim, the first Afghan anesthetist, was also trained at FMIC by French specialists, and at Chennai Cardiac Center.

Najeeb worked full time for two years at FMIC as the Head of Cardiovascular Surgery. His accomplishments were extraordinary.

His story demonstrates both the promise and the obstacle to re-building Afghanistan's systems. The promise is that he and his colleagues at FMIC are dedicated to rebuilding their nation. They have tremendous motivation and capacity to learn and practice at international standards. The obstacle is that Afghanistan is an uncertain and unstable environment and families must make decisions in their own best interests.

Najeeb left his full-time position at FMIC in January 2012. He is not married and most members of his immediate and extended family live outside Afghanistan, some in the U.S., the U.K., and Australia. His brother and two sisters live in Germany. When his father retired from the Army he joined them. Since then he divides his time between Europe and Kabul. While he has committed to work at FMIC for six months each year, he often spends more time there than that.

La Chaîne agreed to increase the number of its mission teams to compensate for Najeeb's decreased presence at FMIC, and the pediatric cardiac surgery team at AKUH, in Karachi, agreed to conduct some missions. With these arrangements, Afghan children will continue to have uninterrupted in-country access to sophisticated cardiac surgery. It is, however, a setback in terms of building Afghan capacity. Najeeb's story highlights the fragility of maintaining sophisticated programs in Afghanistan. Nobody ever said it would be easy.

Dr. Rahima

One of Najeeb's closest professional colleagues in FMIC's cardiac program is Dr. Rahima Stanekzai, chief of the cardiology service. Like Najeeb, her subspecialty training, in both pediatric and adult cardiology, was in France. Rahima defies the western stereotype of Afghan women. She is a wife, a mother, and she has a successful career in medicine. She was the first, and remains the only, female cardiologist in Afghanistan.

Rahima is Pashtun. She was born in 1968 in Logar Province. She was one of nine children in her family. She and her husband, Muhammad Zafar, have three children, ages thirteen, ten, and four. Muhammad Zafar studied pharmacy at Kabul University and he now works as a pharmacist at a private clinic in Kabul.

During the Mujahidin civil war, Rahima lived with her family in Kabul. Those were difficult times for her. "During the war there were catastrophes. On some days there were as many as 3,000 rocket attacks in Kabul. I worked at Jumhoriat Hospital. Injured people were brought there and put in a big hall. Always when I came to work I checked to see if any of my brothers or sisters was there. That's why I seem older than my age. I will never forget."

When the Taliban took power, her situation actually improved. They forbade her from working at Jumhoriat Hospital because both men and women were treated there, so she moved to Rabia Balki, one of Kabul's largest maternity hospitals. The Taliban didn't object to women working there.

Her experience at Rabia Balki was satisfying and rewarding. She held a faculty appointment at Kabul Medical University and taught students. She rose to be director of the hospital and held that position for two years. "For women it was not difficult to work at Rabia Balki. It was good work for me. I know there were lots of problems for students and for women. They weren't able to work outside. But for me it was okay."

After the Taliban were routed from power in 2001, Rahima was approached by representatives from the French Embassy to go to France and be trained in adult cardiology. From 2002 to 2004, she studied at the *Centre Hospitalier Sud Francilien*, near Paris. In 2004, she received a certificate in adult cardiology from Versailles Medical University and became a member of the French Society of Cardiology. Upon returning to Afghanistan, she became a lecturer at Kabul Medical University.

Rahima was recruited to work at FMIC in 2005. "At that time the construction was just completed. I saw my first child patient in a clinic with Prof. Alain Deloche. Because of his encouragement, I decided to change my practice from adult to pediatric cardiology and, in 2006, I went again to France to study." She studied for one month with Prof. Daniel Sidi, a vice president of La Chaîne and head of cardiology at the famous Paris children's hospital, *Hôpital Necker-Enfants Malades*. Now she returns to France each year to continue her studies under Prof. Sidi and to participate in international conferences. She has received additional training on-site at FMIC by French cardiologists visiting with mission teams.

Rahima says FMIC stands out from all Afghan hospitals. "Just look at the intensive care unit. There is no comparable place like it in any other hospital in Afghanistan. Most of our people cannot send their children abroad for care. Now they can come here. Children with very critical conditions can now be treated in Afghanistan and they survive. This is not possible in another hospital. FMIC is a revolution, especially for pediatric cardiology and pediatric cardiac surgery."

Rahima conducts continuing medical education sessions for

doctors at other hospitals, both in Kabul and elsewhere in Afghanistan. She believes it is FMIC's obligation to share the knowledge of its doctors as much as possible. "I do sessions on different pediatric cardiology cases. Doctors are interested to attend our sessions. FMIC is the first hospital that does this in the country."

She told me a story that exemplifies her commitment to work and her career. "After I had started work at FMIC I went to Eric and Kate and told them that I needed time off the next day. Kate asked 'Why tomorrow?' I said 'Because it will be time for my caesarian section.' Eric was alarmed. He said, 'Oh! Then why are you working today? In France, mothers take one month maternity leave before a C-section.' I had my C-section the next day and started work again fifteen days later. I have to work."

Rahima's husband, Muhammad Zafar, supports her in her career. "When I first went to France, my second child was just one year old. When I was in France he took responsibility for the children. There is no problem for me with my family. He helps me a lot at home."

Rahima is both optimistic and contemplative about what will happen when international military forces withdraw from Afghanistan in 2014. "It is difficult to say what will happen in the future. FMIC is a hospital. Every kind of government has a need for a hospital. FMIC should continue to develop in any case. People need doctors and treatment."

YOGANA AND HER NURSES

Yogana, daughter of Mohammad Obaid, was admitted to FMIC in October 2011. Alex Leis was very involved in her care. During one of my visits to Kabul, shortly after Yogana's admission in late 2011, he took me to the ward to meet Yogana and her parents.

Yogana was lying in bed, breathing with the aid of a respirator. Her only visible movement was her eyes. Her gaze briefly followed me to the side of her bed where her parents stood. They were a well-dressed and handsome couple. Alex introduced me and they both greeted me warmly.

Alex gave me some background on Yogana's case. "Before the onset of symptoms she was a healthy seven-year-old child and developing normally. Her first symptom was a sore throat and then she developed a fever."

Muhammad Obaid nodded in agreement. "She was very happy. She never had serious health problems," he added. "We thought she had a cold. We took her to a local doctor who tried to treat her symptoms, but he did not diagnose her main problem."

"Very soon her situation changed for the worse," Alex said, "and it quickly became quite dramatic. She developed paralysis in her legs and then it began affect other parts of her body."

By now the family was desperately trying to get care for Yogana. "We took her to other hospitals, but they could do nothing for her," Mohammad Obaid said. "Finally we took her to Indira Gandhi Hospital."

Her condition progressed so rapidly that, after a short time, she was paralyzed to the point that she could not breathe and she had an episode of cardiac arrest. "The doctors at Indira Gandhi said she should be brought to FMIC immediately," Alex said. "They know this is the only place in Afghanistan where an intensive care unit exists. Her condition was life threatening by the time she got here. Her blood pressure fluctuated from very high to very low and her heart rate was extremely fast. Soon she was completely paralyzed and unable to move anything except her eyes. She was placed on a ventilator to assist her breathing. Despite her paralysis, she was awake and conscious. She was looking around and was extremely anxious."

Tests revealed that Yogana had Guillain-Barré Syndrome, a neurologic disease that disrupts the immune system and causes degeneration of peripheral nerves. GBS is a serious disease that requires immediate hospitalization because of the rapid rate at which it worsens. The sooner appropriate treatment is started the better the chance of a good outcome. The disease can be life-threatening if weakness spreads to muscles that control breathing, heart rate, and blood pressure. The prognosis in developed countries – where diagnosis can be made quickly, where appropriate treatment can be started promptly, and where effective rehabilitation can be implemented – is that eighty to eight-five percent of cases will have complete recovery; ten percent will have permanent neurological damage; and about five percent will die. The prognosis is much poorer in Afghanistan where optimal conditions don't exist.

With the ability to diagnose Yogana's condition, FMIC doctors started treatment. This involved administering polyvalent immunoglobulin. The goal was to achieve immunomodulation, or adjustment of her immune response to a desired level. But this early pharmaceutical step was just the beginning. The medical part of Yogana's treatment only occurred for a few days. Immunomodulation had to be accompanied by significant supportive care or serious long-term complications could occur. She required constant massage and manipulation of her limbs, or she would never have full function of them again, and she was at high risk of getting bed sores that could lead to serious infection. It was critical that an active exercise therapy program be carried out. Rehabilitation and nursing care were now the priority.

"We are very pleased and grateful for Yogana's care at FMIC," Mohammad Obaid said. "We didn't know about FMIC before Yogana got sick. My brother told us we should come here because this is the best hospital in all of Afghanistan. We didn't at first, but we should have. The doctor in charge of intensive care, Amena, works very hard every night and every day; even in the middle of the night she comes if necessary. All the doctors, including Dr. Alex, and the nurses work very hard."

Alex smiled at Mohammad Obaid's compliment. "Dr. Alex tells me that you and your wife are very involved in Yogana's care," I said. "What do you do for her?"

"We spend almost all our time at FMIC. About four times every day and night we move her legs and arms. Now she can breathe better, eat some, and even speak. Her arms are not working, but she can move her fingers and she can shake her legs some."

I thanked the family for allowing me to meet Yogana and gave them my best wishes for her complete recovery. I knew it would be long and uncertain. FMIC didn't have a proper physical therapy department, but the nurses had good experience caring for post-operative orthopedic and neurosurgical cases; despite that, a lot of her recovery would depend on her parents, both in the hospital and at home.

A few weeks later, while I was back in the States, I exchanged emails with Alex and asked him how Yogana's recovery had been. "It's been great," he replied. "Her progress was steady and successful. She quickly became able to breathe without assistance of a respirator and, after a month, she started to eat without being fed by a gastric tube. She always knew what was going on around her and she started to make comments on what services she liked and what ones she didn't like."

I was delighted to hear such a positive report.

"She has gone home now," he continued. "In fact, I saw her just yesterday for a follow-up visit. She can move her legs much better now; she can stand with help and she can sit alone. She has gained weight. That's a very positive development. Her parents are extremely happy and thankful for her recovery. I took a picture of them. They asked that I send it to you. They send their warmest greetings to you and thank you for your support."

I couldn't have been happier. That kind of feedback is why I love the work I do with FMIC, not that I had anything to do with Yogana's recovery.

Yogana's successful recovery would not have been possible without good nursing care. At one of my hospitals in the U.S., I apparently wasn't recognizing my nursing staff as much as my vice president of nursing thought I should be. She told me: "Lee, let's be clear about what goes on in hospitals."

I was pretty sure I knew what went on in hospitals. After all, I had a master's degree in hospital management and many years' experience running them. Nevertheless, I knew enough to defer to my VP of nursing. "Okay," I said, "what goes on in hospitals?"

"Nursing care goes on in hospitals, Lee. Doctors come and doctors go, but nurses are on-site caring for patients around the clock every day."

That was good advice in the U.S. and it is just as relevant in Afghanistan. We recognized from the beginning that the paucity of skilled Afghan nurses, especially females, would be a bigger obstacle to expanding services and delivering quality care at FMIC than the availability of physicians and surgeons.

Nursing is a fragile profession in Afghanistan. Nationally, the number of nurses is grossly deficient. In 2011, the World Health Organization reported that Afghanistan had five nurses per 10,000 population. Only twelve out of 175 countries reported on by WHO had fewer nurses per capita than Afghanistan. By comparison, France had eighty nurses per 10,000 population, the U.S. had ninety-five, Canada had 101, and the U.K. had 128. Ireland topped all with 195. An issue just as important as the overall shortage of nurses is the paltry number of female nurses in Afghanistan. A 2011 Afghanistan government report stated that only fifteen percent of nurses and nurses' assistants in the country are female.

Both the French and AKU contribute to developing a strong Afghan nursing service at FMIC. The outstanding and dedicated French nurses who accompanied surgical teams on short-term missions introduced their Afghan counterparts to international best practices, and long-term French volunteers remained in Kabul for months working side-by-side with them. However, much of the credit for capacity development of Afghan nurses at FMIC belongs to the AKU nursing leaders assigned to Kabul from Karachi. Nursing has been one of AKU's premier academic programs and services since the University's inception. the School of Nursing was the first academic program offered at AKU. For more than two decades, it has been a leader in nursing education and research in Pakistan and the developing world.

Afghan nurses have steadily moved up to replace expatriate nurses in leadership positions at FMIC. At the end of 2005, FMIC's entire nursing team consisted of a nursing administrator assigned from AKUH, Karachi, one French nurse, and ten Afghan nurses. At the end of 2012, FMIC's nursing team consisted of 115 Afghans and six international nurses – one Tajik and five Pakistanis. Of the Afghan nurses, eighty were male and thirty-five were female. That wasn't a bad ratio for Afghanistan, but not close to what we eventually wanted. The international nurses mainly held administrative and teaching positions. Most patient care was done by Afghan nurses. French nurses still visited FMIC with surgical mission teams, but far less frequently than in the past. By early 2013, national nurses held head nurse positions in four of FMIC's five nursing units.

I have special regard for all the nurses at FMIC. Their courage and gumption is impressive. Like all Afghans, during decades of war they and their families have suffered injury and death and they, too, have been intimidated and terrorized by warlords and the Taliban. The women especially have faced cultural and gender bigotry. This adversity hasn't deterred them from their personal and professional ambitions. They are as feisty and self-assured as any of their male peers. A couple of good examples are Asma Nouri and Nazila Hussain.

"I wanted to be a doctor but my family didn't have enough money," Asma told me. She works in the intensive care unit and is one of the few Afghan nurses who obtained a Bachelor of Science in Nursing (BScN) degree from Kabul Medical University. The curriculum there was developed with consulting assistance of AKU's School of Nursing. "When I started school, people laughed at the idea that a nurse would go to school for four years. When I graduated, I really wanted to work at FMIC. Other hospitals all have problems, especially in nursing. They have no respect for nurses. Nurses don't have good reputations in Afghanistan. I love my job at FMIC and I like to be working here. My family came here and found that my situation was good and now they support me."

Nazila, who also works in the intensive care unit, agrees with Asma. "My big sister is a doctor, but I wanted to be a nurse," she said. "During the Taliban period all the females had to stay at home. The only ones who could work were nurses and doctors. That's why I wanted to be a nurse. At first my family was not happy with me, but slowly, slowly they became happier and now they are completely happy. I am married now and I have a child. My husband also supports me working at FMIC."

A few weeks after my email exchange with Alex, I was back in Kabul. During a meeting with some of the nurses I asked them if they remembered Yogana. I said I was amazed at her successfully recovery and that I understood that her nursing care was as important, if not more important, than her medical treatment.

"Of course we remember her," said Rauf Sayed Hashimi, an instructor in FMIC's Nursing Education Services. "We all remember her well. The government hospital couldn't care for her. Her father came to us and asked for her to be admitted. He was crying. We didn't have any beds available in the intensive care unit, but we talked with the doctors and we shifted a patient to the ward so we could admit her."

Laila Khymani, the AKU nurse assigned as the senior administrator of the nursing division and the hospital's quality assurance program described the requirements for Yogana's successful rehabilitation. "She was in a debilitated state. It was important to not overwork her muscles or that would have increased her weakness. Our nurses began a daily regimen of range of motion exercises for her. Her parents worked side-by-side with us and we taught them how to exercise her. Her mother is a teacher. At night she stayed with Yogana and in the mornings she went to school. Her father is a plumber but he spent so much time caring for Yogana that he was unable to work during this time."

Laila summed up Yogana's case in a way that reminded me of my former VP of nursing's advice. I guess it truly – and appropriately – reflects the way nurses see their role. "Sometimes in these kinds of cases the medical care reaches status quo. There is nothing more medicine can do. The doctors have done all they can, but nursing care never ends. Nurses have to do suctioning every two hours, give medications right on time, bathe the patient, keep them comfortable … everything. That can never end. Nursing care requires a lot of persistence and dedication, without losing hope, whatever the outcome may be."

Yogana's departure from the hospital was celebrated by the staff and her family. She was lavishly dressed and taken home in a car filled with flowers. Her parents said this was done because this day began Yogana's second life.

"When patients get discharged," Laila said, "their parents some-times give the nurses a card for having done a good job. Yogana's mother gave me a card I took a picture of and keep in my mobile phone because I don't want to lose track of it. It said 'God sure listens, understands and knows the hope and fears you keep in your heart for when you trust in his love, miracles happen.' She wrote this for the whole team of nursing. I kept this for the memory."

Laila should keep the card Yogana's mother gave her because FMIC's nurses are part of the miracles that happen there.

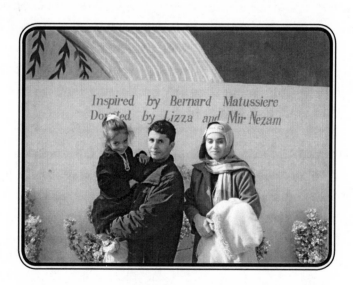

Yogana with her parents

The total charges for Yogana's seventy-three days of care were US$10,212.00. The family paid US$2,040.00 and the hospital patient welfare program covered US$8,172.00, or eighty percent.

FOUNDATIONS
OF SUCCESS

There is ongoing discussion in the United States about the lack of success of international development and reconstruction efforts in Afghanistan. Multiple studies and investigations have found that projects totaling billions of dollars have not been successful. While the causes of failure are many, common themes have been lack of adequate oversight of contractors resulting in poor quality outcomes, and lack of adequate training and preparation of Afghans to sustain the projects. With their withdrawal of military forces, many western governments have committed billions more to be invested toward new development initiatives. Due to uncertain security, the likelihood of more responsible oversight of projects is no more likely than it was for the past decade. The unfortunate result may be withholding of committed development funds. This will be to the substantial detriment of the Afghan people and to the eventual security and stability of the region.

After more than eight years of existence, the FMIC represents a successful model that should be considered – and possibly emulated – by others as a means of ensuring successful development outcomes. Its foundations of success are straightforward and simple. They are few, hence, they are easy to keep track of, and on the surface the partners all agree to them, but as the saying goes, 'the devil is in the details.' The ingredients of FMIC's success include: a unique four-party public-private-partnership that spreads both obligation and risk among the partners; a well-crafted Memorandum of Agreement that clearly states the obligations of each partner; a good governance process; an unyielding commitment to quality; ensuring beneficiaries' financial and physical access to the institution; pursuit of financial sustainability; and an emphasis on Afghan capacity development.

The rules of engagement for FMIC's partnership are set forth in its Memorandum of Agreement. That agreement, negotiated over more than a year and signed at the inauguration ceremony on April 8, 2006, is the centerpiece of the extraordinary partnership. It is not a document that gathers dust on the shelf. It is a living document, constantly referred to by the partners as a reminder of their commitments to one another and to the institution. Not all of the commitments have been met but, in eight years – and under extraordinarily challenging circumstances – the partners have all done a remarkable job of living up to them.

Another important contributor to FMIC's success has been the governance process. Good governance is a critical ingredient of any organization's success. This is especially true in the case of one as complex as FMIC, with four partners – two government and two private. FMIC management definitely needs support of a good board to guide it and to back it up when necessary. FMIC's Memorandum of Agreement stipulates that the chairman of the board is appointed by the AKDN. I have been privileged to serve as chair since FMIC's inauguration in 2006.

FMIC's board has eight members, including five from the AKDN, one from the Government of Afghanistan, and two from the

French parties -- Enfants Afghans and La Chaîne. A representative of the French Embassy in Afghanistan routinely participates on an *ex officio* basis. Through 2013, twenty-four board meetings were held, nearly all on-site in Kabul. The dedication of members to their duties has been remarkable. Despite occasional periods of instability and security advisories, hardly any member, including attendees from the French Embassy, has ever missed a meeting.

Members of FMIC's management and clinical staff and its doctors and nurses are routinely invited to board meetings. As chairman, I have tried to use the board as a forum for learning. It has been a setting to demonstrate, by example, to the Government of Afghanistan and our Afghan colleagues what constitutes good governance and why that is important in institutional leadership. We have sought to operate with the highest integrity and transparency. Meetings are conducted with respect for all points of view and input by all partners. Issues have almost always been resolved with consensus and without need for formally counting votes.

A critical element that sets FMIC apart from all other hospitals in Afghanistan is the quality of its services. There was consensus from the beginning to pursue the highest possible quality. FMIC's mission statement says it will "provide exemplary quality and safe care to patients." That sounds simple, and it is easy to put on paper, but it is difficult to achieve, especially in the difficult operating environment the hospital faces in Afghanistan.

As FMIC refined its approach to quality it continued to raise its performance bar. Whenever possible it adopted international standards for clinical care. It offered itself as a new standard in Afghanistan and a model for others to pursue. On April 29,

2009, in just its third year of operations, FMIC was awarded ISO 9001:2008 certification following a vigorous independent audit by a European-based auditor. ISO certification is a global benchmark providing assurance about an organization's ability to satisfy quality requirements and to enhance customer satisfaction. With this recognition, FMIC became the first healthcare institution in Afghanistan to be endorsed by an international agency for providing high quality services. That an Afghanistan hospital could achieve this was a source of great pride for the entire country. The award ceremony held on May 28, 2009, was attended by approximately 500 guests including His Excellency the Minister of Public Health Dr. Syed Mohammad Amin Fatimi, and other guests from government, the public and private hospital sectors, and embassies. Since its initial certification, FMIC has repeatedly been recertified with no non-conformance findings.

In February 2011, as part of its fifth anniversary celebration, FMIC held its first International Pediatric Symposium. This was the first such event ever held in Afghanistan. FMIC's staff, both physicians and nurses, presented case studies from their practices. Presentations were also made by physicians from the U.S., Spain, Pakistan, and Canada. This event inspired me as much as any anything FMIC had accomplished during its existence. I sensed that FMIC had moved beyond just delivering the highest quality health care in the country and it was now contributing to nation building. Approximately 230 participants attended from nine countries. The pride of FMIC's Afghan staff was palpable. They realized they could host an event of interest to the international community and that their experiences and accomplishments were of interest to health care professionals from around the globe. Follow-on symposia were held in 2012 and 2013. Despite security incidents that complicated international attendance, local interest throughout Afghanistan has continued to grow. In 2013, ninety-six papers were submitted for presentation and approximately 500 individuals attended the event, the highest number to date. We decided a larger venue would have to be found for the 2014 program.

Another important quality-focused event initiated and hosted by FMIC has been its annual Quality Improvement and Patient Safety Convention. This program features projects – conducted by FMIC's medical, nursing, and allied health staffs – focused on improvement in quality care. It serves as a model for other providers in the community by demonstrating practical and doable steps they can take to improve quality in their hospitals. Like the International Symposia, local interest in this event has grown each year. In November 2013, Her Excellency, Suraya Dalil, the Minister of Public Health, was the chief guest speaker. Approximately 200 individuals attended, including many from public and private hospitals throughout Kabul.

The most ambitious quality management strategy undertaken by FMIC to date is its pursuit of accreditation by the Joint Commission International (JCI), a U.S.-based accreditation body that is the gold standard in the world. JCI standards are rigorous and difficult to comply with. The FMIC team is being assisted in its preparation for JCI accreditation by AKUH, Karachi. FMIC must overcome many obstacles to be JCI accredited, but the effort alone has its rewards by expanding the staff's insight and knowledge about what constitutes the highest standard of care.

FMIC's mission statement says its services will be both *financially* and *physically* accessible to patients with limited means to pay. There are Afghan patients who can afford to pay for good quality medical care. That is demonstrated by the fact that many go abroad for care, bearing the cost of both transportation and hospitalization. Nevertheless, Afghanistan is one of the poorest countries in the world and most patients cannot pay the full or, often, even partial costs of their services. FMIC receives payment for its services in local currency but purchases nearly all of its medical equipment and most of its supplies on the international market, using international currency – usually U.S. dollars or Euros. Because its services are, in nearly every case, the best available in Afghanistan, it sets its prices at or near the top of what other providers in the market charge for services. Clearly, patients who have limited means to pay can't afford to pay this amount and, therefore, require assistance.

At the outset of FMIC's existence, a patient welfare program was established. As the financiers of FMIC, the partners realized they did not have limitless capacity to fund free or subsidized care. FMIC is a private institution and it was not intended to supplant the public sector's responsibility to provide free care for Afghan citizens. While the hospital's vision includes being financially *accessible*, it also includes becoming a financially *sustainable* institution. There is obviously tension between those two visions. If the hospital's funding requirements exceed the partners' capacity, they will either have to reduce the amount of welfare or reduce services.

A system to assess families' ability to pay was implemented – a form of *means test*. That was not easy in Afghanistan but, over the years, it has worked effectively. In FMIC's first year of existence over one-half million dollars of patient welfare was provided -- this constituted thirty-nine percent of the hospital's total revenue. Most of that supported patients getting complex inpatient care.

To support access to care for needy patients, the Government of Afghanistan committed US$1 million dollars for patient welfare each year. This was in addition to the private partners' contribution. During the period from early 2006 through September 2013, FMIC provided approximately US$18,470,000 worth of patient welfare support to over a quarter-million patients. This accounted for approximately thirty-five percent of all patient revenue, more than sixty-two percent of inpatients, and about sixteen percent of outpatients. Patients from every one of Afghanistan's thirty-four provinces have received support from the patient welfare program.

Ensuring patients' financial access to care at FMIC is only part of the challenge. Ensuring their physical access is no less a challenge. Limited physical access to health care is a national problem. One reason is the scarce availability and poor distribution of the nation's health providers. In 2012, WHO reported there were only two physicians and five nurses available for every 10,000 population. Another reason is the population's geographic isolation. Afghanistan's mountains pose some of the most rugged terrain in the world. Much of the population lives in areas where roads barely exist and weather conditions are often extreme. Finally, there is the effect of seemingly endless war. Health facilities are sometimes destroyed, health workers are killed or threatened, and the risk of passage through hostile areas is just one more impediment to travel facing patients and their families.

E-Health technology, also called telemedicine, can transcend mountains and long distances and seems to be an ideal technology for Afghanistan. FMIC is privileged to have a unique enabling partner to help pursue this initiative. Roshan, the AKDN telecommunications company operating in Afghanistan, has contributed its technical expertise and influence in the global telecommunications industry to make FMIC a forerunner in e-Health in the region. FMIC launched Afghanistan's first e-Health link connecting FMIC to AKUH, Karachi in March 2007. The first application was tele-radiology. FMIC had limited radiology resources at that time. AKUH, Karachi made initial readings and gave second opinions on x-ray exams done at FMIC. The project was funded by Roshan, and equipment and software was provided by Cisco Systems, International.

In a speech inaugurating the network, Nadeem Khan anticipated that FMIC's e-Health program would eventually be expanded to include tele-pathology and live patient consultations in clinics – and it would even connect Kabul with Bamyan. All that happened and even more. Today, FMIC's e-Health facilities link five countries: Afghanistan, Pakistan, Kenya, Tajikistan, and France. Linkages exist between four cities in Afghanistan: Kabul, Bamyan, Faizabad, and Kandahar. Steps are now being taken to create links with remote health centers in the provinces of Badakhshan and Bamyan. This will extend FMIC's e-Health consultation services and e-Learning training sessions to Afghan staff and patients in even more remote areas. As of December 2013, since FMIC first launched its e-Health initiative in 2007, it has provided approximately 11,300 e-Health consultations to Afghan patients.

It's not an exaggeration to say that the AKDN operates one of the most effective e-Health systems in the developing world. The network now encompasses e-Health and e-Learning. In the future, it is planned to implement m-Health, the use of mobile phones to provide support health workers in the field and for data collection. As good as the network is, there are major issues to be overcome, not the least of which is cost. The World Health

Organization defines e-Health as a "cost-effective use of information and communications technologies in support of health and health-related fields. . . ." Whether or not e-Health is cost-effective is debatable. It depends on what it's being compared to: compared to patients having no access to care; or compared to reliance on alternative, even more costly solutions to provide care? FMIC is demonstrating that e-Health can dramatically improve a populations' access to quality care, but the technology is expensive and people in Afghanistan are poor. As a result, the network cannot pay for itself. FMIC has been fortunate until now to have Roshan and other partners -- including French and Canadian development agencies -- to underwrite the initiative. Ways must be identified to generate income surpluses in order to offset e-Health losses, otherwise, ongoing donors will have to be found to fund the system. This is not an issue unique to FMIC and the AKDN. It is one facing anyone trying to implement this extremely relevant technology anyplace in the developing world.

AFGHAN CAPACITY
DEVELOPMENT

The partners all agree that FMIC's mission to provide exemplary and high quality care is important. That is unquestioned. The Memorandum of Agreement left no doubt that the essential purpose of the Mother and Child Hospital is the delivery of ". . . improved services for the prevention and treatment of diseases and conditions affecting the health and well-being of Afghan mothers and children . . . ." Stories about FMIC's successes in healing and saving the lives of sick and injured Afghan children abound. FMIC has set the standard for delivery of high quality health care of an international level.

FMIC has another important purpose. The Memorandum of Agreement also addresses training Afghans. Increasing the capacity of Afghan doctors, nurses, and other health professionals is understood to be as important, if not more important, than the service mission. A June 2012 Ministry of Public Health report proposed a national priority program entitled *Health for All Afghans*. The report concluded that, "There is a lack of both qualified, skilled health care workers across a wide range of specialties and training programs to expand the core basic health services."

Miracles can be helped to happen by hard work, preparation, and

185

persistence. The partners at FMIC have devoted considerable resources and effort to training and mentoring Afghan health professionals. Doctors, nurses, technicians, and others have been sent
abroad for training, and scores of French and Pakistani staff and
volunteers have conducted training for Afghans in Kabul.

Implicit in the Mother and Child Hospital and FMIC models
of Afghan capacity development were La Chaîne-sponsored mission teams. The mission doctors are extraordinarily dedicated to
humanitarian service, not only in Afghanistan, but in other war-
torn and poor countries around the world. They have worked
in Vietnam, Cambodia, Sri Lanka, Indonesia, Senegal, Haiti,
Palestine, East Timor, Egypt, Morocco, Russia, and the Ukraine.
They cared for civilians in Bagdad during the Second Gulf War
and in Haiti after the earthquake.

From 2005 until March 2013, thirty-four physicians and surgeons made 195 mission visits to Kabul. Each visit spanned a
few weeks in length. The mission teams work side-by-side with
Afghan doctors, nurses, and technicians, teaching them advanced
surgical and medical techniques. Most mission doctors are French
nationals but some are Pakistani, Spanish, German, Canadian,
and American. A few are Afghan expatriates living in Europe and
North America. Some are retired, but many are in active practice and at the peak of their careers. Nearly all have experience at
prestigious academic centers. Their specialties include the whole
gamut of medical, surgical, and diagnostic areas. Specialty nurses,
operating theater technicians, and perfusionists are also members
of the teams.

During FMIC's short history, the amount of training provided
to Afghans is impressive. From 2006 through 2013, nearly 560

training opportunities were provided outside Afghanistan to all categories of staff including doctors, nurses, allied health, engineering and technical, and support and administrative. Training locations included academic centers in France, India, Japan, Belgium, and at AKU in Karachi. Most training for non-medical staff has been at AKUH, Karachi but, whenever possible, training is delivered in Afghanistan. Nurses have been given instruction in clinical practice areas and have also been trained for leadership roles as shift supervisors, unit head nurses, and clinical care team leaders.

Allied Health staff received technical training in pharmacy, laboratory, and advance imaging areas such as general radiology, CT scan, and MRI. Technical training was given to staff in plant maintenance and biomedical engineering. Administrative and support staff were trained in finance and materials management; information technology, hospital information systems, and telemedicine; human resources; laundry management; and cooking hygiene and kitchen maintenance. Those who required it were taught effective writing and oral presentation skills.

Some Afghan staff members have been trained in conflict resolution. Decades of war and conflict have created a culture characterized by aggression, intimidation, and fear. Unfortunately, those behaviors sometimes rear their ugly heads inside FMIC's walls. Self-appointed big shots, accustomed to getting what they want by throwing their weight around, frequently bully the hospital's doctors, nurses, and security guards. Ethnic rivalries sometimes erupt and tempers flare. Such behavior is common in Afghanistan's institutions, including its hospitals, but it cannot be tolerated at FMIC. It is essential that FMIC maintain good order and a gentle, caring environment, not only for its patients and families, but also for the sake of its staff; hence, training in conflict resolution is important.

FMIC's e-Learning program has enabled its staff to train Afghan health workers beyond Kabul, in Bamyan, Faizabad, and Kandahar. More than 3,200 Afghan staff in those provinces have benefitted from e-Learning sessions. The beauty of this training is that the benefit of initial training of FMIC staff by the partners is now cascading. Many of the e-Learning sessions are accomplished by Afghans training other Afghans. The same is true for the many continuing medical and nursing programs now conducted by FMIC's Afghan physicians and nurses for their colleagues in Kabul and elsewhere in the country.

In 2008, the French Development Agency (AFD) awarded a grant of two million Euros to the Aga Khan Foundation to develop human resources at FMIC through the year 2011. The project was titled "Strengthening Human Resources for Health at FMIC". The main objective was "contributing to the reduction of mortality and morbidity rates in children by enabling the strengthening of human resources." The Aga Khan Foundation commissioned an external evaluation to measure the project's results. The evaluator concluded that, "Overall the project achieved beyond expectations." More Afghans were trained than originally planned, and services were able to be expanded at FMIC with a decreased number of expatriates and medical missions.

International donors readily fund programs at the primary care level, especially programs focused on maternal and child care. Studies have found that the quality of Afghanistan's basic health services has improved significantly in recent years, resulting in a significant decrease in infant mortality. The potential dollar-for-dollar population health gains from investments in primary care initiatives are persuasive. In contrast, international donors do not readily fund the delivery of secondary and tertiary care, because of its perceived high cost and drain on scarce available resources in poor countries. At the same time, the worldwide prevalence of chronic, non-communicable diseases, as well as heart disease and cancer -- previously thought to be problems mainly among wealthier populations -- can no longer be ignored.

The Ministry of Public Health acknowledges that little attention has been given to secondary and tertiary care. According to the 2004 Afghanistan National Hospital Survey, compared to other developing countries with similar levels of income, Afghanistan has a relatively low number of hospitals and hospital beds. The ratio of one bed per 1,000 people, recommended by the World Health Organization, has not been met across the country, including Kabul.

In June 2010, the Kabul Medical University and AKU jointly authored a paper on postgraduate medical education in Afghanistan. They concluded that the specialty and subspecialty training or physicians is vital for improvement of the Afghan health system. The Government of Afghanistan operates postgraduate medical education training programs in Afghanistan. Around 200 medical graduates are selected annually for training in twenty-one medical specialties. The majority, more than ninety percent, are trained in Ministry of Public Health-managed public-sector hospitals. Unfortunately, the quality of these programs is poor. The curricula are very out of date, many programs have little to no didactic training, and clinical supervision is poor – sometimes non-existent.

Afghans who have the means to get care in other countries do so. The lack of good quality specialized medical services within Afghanistan has created significant community dissatisfaction with the health sector, and results in thousands of patients seeking healthcare abroad. In addition to the costs of care, this adds the further burden of costs for transportation and housing. It is estimated that Afghanistan loses US$80 million per year due to the lack of availability of quality hospital services in the country.

One of FMIC's most important Afghan capacity development initiatives has been that of postgraduate medical education. The dire reality is that competent specialists simply do not exist in specialty areas that are critical to the basic delivery of good medical care, especially pathology, radiology, and anesthesia. Moreover, there are no oversight bodies to ensure that physicians practice within their competency levels, based on formal training. This places the public at great risk.

With start-up funding provided by the Canadian International Development Agency, FMIC began a postgraduate medical education program in April 2012. The curricula were developed by AKU's College of Medicine in collaboration with the Ministry of Public Health. Six residents started four-year training programs, three each in the specialties of Pediatric Surgery and Pediatric Medicine. In April 2013, seventeen more residents -- including a second class in surgery and medicine, and additional specialties of Radiology, Pathology, Orthopedics, Anesthesiology, and Cardiology -- were admitted for training. Future residents in Obstetrics and Gynecology are planned in preparation to operate the new high-risk maternal unit. These residencies are all critical to FMIC's success, even its existence. It is already a functioning tertiary hospital, offering the highest levels of care in Afghanistan, but its specialist staffing is extremely thin. As programs are expanded beyond the existing mother and child components, to become a more comprehensive medical center serving adults in other services, postgraduate medical education will remain a critical element. As AKU's experience in other developing countries has shown, well-trained graduates filter beyond FMIC, into the community, and begin to influence the quality of care there.

OPPORTUNITIES
AND ISSUES

FMIC has many positive things going for it at this point in its short history, not the least of which is recognition of its high quality care and contributions to Afghanistan by patients and their families and by Afghan government officials. In her remarks opening FMIC's Second International Pediatric Conference in 2012, Dr. Suraya Dalil, the Minister of Public Health, said "FMIC has achieved many successes and achieved excellence in many fields in healthcare in Afghanistan. This Institute is a true example of a successful public-private partnership."

Dr. Abdullah Fahim was formerly the Government of Afghanistan's representative on FMIC's governing body and a senior advisor to the Minister of Public Health. He finds it remarkable that Afghans are now able to independently do pediatric cardiac surgery at FMIC. "More than that, not only does FMIC offer high quality services, but it conducts research activities and hosts international conferences. That is not easy to do in Afghanistan. It is a tremendous lesson for our hospitals. We have never before seen this kind of activity in Afghanistan. I hope the leadership of our hospitals follow this example."

New developments are underway that bode well for FMIC's

future. Despite the uncertainties about security in Afghanistan, its political environment, or its economy, the partners have tangibly reaffirmed their long-term commitment to it. In October 2012, a foundation stone-laying ceremony was held to launch construction of a new sixty-six bed facility next to the existing eighty-five bed children's hospital. The foundation stone was laid by Monsieur Laurent Fabius, the French Minister of Foreign Affairs. The ceremony was attended by the vice president of the Islamic Republic of Afghanistan, His Excellency Karim Khalili; and His Highness, The Aga Khan. The French government and His Highness each committed funding grants of €9 million, nearly US$12.5 million. The new facility will house fifty-two obstetrics and gynecology beds for high-risk maternity services and fourteen neonatal intensive care bassinets. La Chaîne's dream of a mother and child hospital in Kabul will finally be realized when the project is completed in early 2015. The new programs will be consistent with national priorities and will make significant contributions to the health of mothers and newborns in Afghanistan. Not only will the hospital provide high quality services, it will feature women's health promotion and disease prevention. Through programs in education and research it can positively influence maternal and child morbidity and mortality in remote and rural areas.

The original Memorandum of Agreement stated that once it was apparent the partnership would be extended beyond its initial three-year term, additional land would be sought for further expansion. The agreement has now been twice renewed and, in October 2012, the Government of Afghanistan granted an additional seventeen acres of land for development of an expanded hospital complex. The additional land is located across a small road leading to the mother and child hospital. The two sites will be connected by newly-constructed corridors. Various program options for the expanded complex are still being explored, but likely plans include an academic health sciences center with education and research programs, operating in partnership with AKU and other universities, and a 250- to 400-bed hospital providing subspecialty care in adult medicine and surgery, mental health, and family medicine. This expansion will be implemented over several years. It will enable the formation of new partnerships with donors to create *service institutes* in areas including cardiac, oncology, orthopedics, neurosciences, and others. It will also enable deepened collaboration with Kabul Medical University and the Ministry of Public Health's Ghazanfar Institute of Health Sciences in postgraduate medical, nursing, and allied health education. It is consistent with the AKDN vision to create a referral center that would be the hub of a cross-border integrated health system encompassing Afghanistan, Northern Pakistan, Tajikistan, and Kyrgyzstan.

Some services have already been located on the new land and plans are underway for others. The Kids' House program, for example, has grown to the extent that La Chaîne wants to relocate it to a larger site. It is only able to serve about 800 families per year in its present location. La Chaîne would like to double that number. Space has been identified on the new land and, hopefully, The Kids' House will be relocated there by the end of 2014.

Much of FMIC's future depends on the state of security in Afghanistan. Neither La Chaîne nor the AKDN are the kind of organizations that run from conflict. To the contrary, they often pursue their humanitarian missions in the midst of it. Nobody knows what will occur when Afghanistan is on its own militarily and is operating under a post-Karzai led government. Will the ethnic and religious factions join together and coexist – perhaps fitfully, but more or less peacefully -- or will they revert to the fighting and destruction of the civil war era? To what extent will Afghanistan's neighboring countries leave it alone or meddle in its affairs in pursuit of their own interests?

Even with international security forces present, the trend for several years has not been encouraging. When I arrived in Kabul in 2004, the country was relatively secure. There were isolated incidences, but Afghans and foreigners were able to travel in the countryside with little risk. Nearly every year since then has seen increased violence and the reemergence of Taliban terrorist activities. Within a year after FMIC's inauguration, Aziz Jan informed the board that the Central Afghanistan region and Kabul were increasingly unstable. He cited frequent rocket attacks around the city, suicide bombings, kidnappings for ransom, and increased criminal activities.

An attack occurred involving one of our own FMIC family in 2011. On January 28 , 2011, Kate Rowlands was injured in a suicide attack while she was shopping at a supermarket in Wazir Akbar Khan, a neighborhood described by some as the "Green Zone" of Kabul – a reference to the safe military and expatriate area in Bagdad. Embassies, offices of large corporations, and NATO headquarters are located in this highly protected area.

During one of my visits to Kabul a few months after the incident, I talked with Kate about it at her home. She said the last thing she expected was to be confronted by a suicide bomber in an upscale supermarket. "Lee, it never crossed my mind. I was just going about my business shopping when all of a sudden it became crazy. I remember hearing 'bang, bang, bang'!"

It happened so fast that at first Kate didn't understand what was happening. "I stupidly thought it was milk bottles falling. Then I saw this poor woman – and this guy. If there was a police I.D. lineup I could still identify him in a minute. He was shooting everywhere. The woman and I were away from everybody else. I first thought 'This is it for this poor lady and me' and then I thought 'No it isn't. It doesn't have to be.' This all went through my mind in a nanosecond. I jumped behind a pillar. The guy was running around and shooting. It was chaos. Next I heard this God Almighty noise and everything went yellow!"

Kate was injured and taken for treatment to the nearby Emergency Hospital – coincidentally, the organization she worked with before she joined FMIC. We were all worried about her and relieved to hear her injuries weren't life-threatening or disabling. "Everybody was incredibly kind to me afterwards," she said. "I came back home and took stock of my life. I thought, 'What do I do, go home to England . . . and then what?' I could sit around and blabber about being in this situation, but Lee, families got killed that day. Four children and their mother and father got killed. I would be extremely selfish if I felt sorry for myself. I decided to put it down to experience and just bloody get on with it."

She found that was easier said than done. "I've been through a lot of situations, but this one took me some time to work through. I had to make myself Kate again. It took some willpower. At first I couldn't even drive and the staff had to pick me up and drive me around. Finally, I pushed myself to get in the car and drive myself."

Where did Kate first go? She went to the place she loved and felt most secure in. "Within a couple of days after the attack I went to

The Kids' House. The families there were incredibly thoughtful and kind to me. They were lovely and so nice. It did me so much good. They took my mind off myself."

Kate said the event had a lasting effect on her. "I reevaluated my life . . . again. Okay, I'm not going to be wonderful and kind overnight and never shout again, but I just don't worry about the small things now. We go around worrying about such small and insignificant things, but we could be gone in one second. I just feel incredibly lucky to be here."

Kate sat quietly for a while. Obviously her mind was someplace else. I waited. After a long drag on her cigarette she said, perhaps more to herself than to me, "Some things are still in the box. The most important things stay in the box."

I don't know if Kate made the connection, but her chosen metaphor of keeping things in a box made me think of the Rwandan nurse who crawled into the box to escape all the death and destruction around her.

The year 2011 continued to be difficult in terms of security. On May 21, a powerful blast occurred at the heavily guarded national military hospital in Kabul, killing six people and injuring more than twenty others. This caused concern at FMIC because it was the first attack we were aware of directed at a hospital. A few weeks later, while the board was in session, we were informed that a suicide attack had occurred at a Ministry of Public Health Comprehensive Health Center in nearby Logar Province. That attack, the second on a health facility within just one month, resulted in thirty-five deaths.

A day later, shortly after midnight on June 25, I was preparing for bed at the Serena Hotel. Suddenly, I heard explosions and artillery fire from somewhere in the distance. It was difficult to tell what area of the city it was coming from. I called Aziz to find out what he knew.

"I just heard from AKDN security that an attack is underway at the Inter-Continental Hotel," he said. "There apparently are many gunmen in the hotel. There are gunfights and ISAF (the international security forces) helicopters are shooting rockets onto the roof."

The Inter-Continental is where I stayed during my first visit to Kabul and I've dined in its restaurant many times since then. It's not far from FMIC. I asked Aziz if everything was okay at the hospital.

"Yes Lee, everything is okay at the hospital and at the staff's residences. Don't worry about anything. I will let you know if there are any new developments."

I didn't sleep much for the rest of the night. Gunfire and explosions went on for hours. By the time it ended the next morning, twenty people were dead, including nine attackers. I remembered the sign I saw at the hotel entrance the first time I stayed there, the one that declared NO WEAPONS.

As the year went on, other attacks occurred in Kabul. A day-long assault at the U.S. Embassy killed nine people; a suicide bomber assassinated Burhanuddin Rabbani; and sectarian violence, mainly Sunni on Shia, resulted in dozens of civilian deaths. The UN said 2011 was the deadliest year on record for Afghan civilians, with 3,021 killed by roadside bombs and suicide attacks.

The FMIC board approved funding for Aziz to upgrade the hospital's security. Safe rooms were constructed at the hospital and at the Pakistani staff guesthouse; additional fencing was erected along the entire hospital boundary wall; closed circuit TV cameras were installed; a vehicle security barrier was installed at the main entry gate; and additional security staff members were hired. While assuring the board that FMIC was taking all necessary steps to guarantee the safety of its patients and staff, Aziz rightfully emphasized that the year had been a difficult one. "Guaranteeing security," he said, "of over 2,500 people on an average day -- including employees, staff, and patient attendants -- is quite a challenge."

As 2012 began, the situation didn't improve. In February, there were violent demonstrations in reaction to the international forces allegedly burning copies of the Quran at a NATO military base. There were riots in March, protesting the alleged murder of sixteen Afghan civilians by a U.S. Army Staff Sergeant; and in April, major attacks were launched on high-profile targets around Kabul including several Western embassies in the heavily-guarded central diplomatic area and the Parliament. On June 2, just one month before I began my trip to a remote area of Badakhshan Province to meet with Salma, a NATO team rescued four medical aid workers who were seized by the Taliban a month earlier. They had been working in flood-stricken parts of the province when they were kidnapped. On July 24, one month after I traveled to Bamyan, three civilians -- including an American engineer -- were shot and killed while driving from Kabul to Bamyan on the Kabul-Bamyan highway.

September was another turbulent month. A suicide bomber detonated explosives near the NATO headquarters in Kabul on

September 8, killing six civilians. The same month, an anti-Islam, American-made movie, posted on YouTube earlier in the year, finally went viral around the Muslim world, causing violent uprisings in Afghanistan and elsewhere. If all of that that wasn't enough, in September, the French satirical magazine, *Charlie Hebdo*, published derogatory cartoons of the Muslim prophet Muhammad. Anticipating Muslim retribution, France closed its embassies and schools in twenty countries, including Afghanistan. This caused special concern at FMIC because of the hospital's well-known French sponsorship. Fortunately, no violence was directed toward the hospital but, just to be safe, French expatriates were sent to Dubai for three days during the worst of the violence in Kabul.

Terrorist attacks in Kabul were comparatively fewer in number during 2013, but an emerging problem was criminal activity, including kidnapping for ransom. Some of FMIC's doctors received threats that members of their families would be kidnapped. That obviously caused distress for them. Because of kidnapping threats directed toward her family, Laila Khymani, FMIC's Director of Nursing, permanently left Kabul and returned to Karachi. The loss of her leadership was a serious setback for FMIC. In August, an AKDN team visiting Bamyan Province was assaulted at gunpoint while traveling on the road from Bamyan City to Band-e-Amir Lake National Park – the same road I traveled on the year before when I visited the five-year-old heart patient, Frishta. The assailants let two of the team go but took the other two as hostages. The motive for the event was thought to be criminal rather than terrorist. Fortunately, after considerable effort by the Afghan government and police, the two hostages were released unharmed.

Due to Taliban efforts to disrupt Afghanistan's presidential elections, 2014 has been a disastrous year, especially for civilians. On

January 17, terrorists attacked La Taverna du Liban, a restaurant located in the Wazir Akbar Khan neighborhood – the same part of town where Kate was injured in an attack. They blew open the front gate and entered the restaurant, firing on all the diners. They killed twenty people, including thirteen international workers, seven Afghans, and the restaurant's owner, Kamel Hamade. La Taverna du Liban was one of my favorite places to dine when I visited Kabul. I had met Kamel Hamade on several occasions. He was a gregarious host who enjoyed interacting with his patrons. When news of the attack broke, I was in Karachi attending a meeting at AKU. Several members of FMIC's management team were with me. They were quite shaken because they had dined in in the restaurant just one night before the attack.

On March 20, two teenage Taliban gunmen sneaked handguns through security at the Serena Hotel. They entered the hotel dining room, and systematically executed nine people, including two children. I knew two of the adults who were killed, both Canadian-Ismailis, followers of the Aga Khan. One of the two that I knew was Zeenab Kassam, a volunteer teaching English to Afghans. I had met her during one of my trips to Kabul; we had both dined in the same dining room where she was later killed.

The other person I knew was Roshan Thomas. I had known Roshan and her husband, Rahim, for nearly twenty years. Roshan was an optometrist and Rahim an ophthalmologist. They worked around the world as volunteers for the AKDN setting up and delivering eye care programs. Rahim helped us set up the eye department at AKU when I was there in the early nineties. Roshan had a special mission in Afghanistan. She worked there for several years, setting up schools, with an emphasis on girls' education.

Before 2014 had hardly started, another senseless killing of a civilian humanitarian worker occurred. Again, it was an event that struck close to home for those of us at FMIC. On April 24, an Afghanistan security guard, employed by CURE International Hospital, shot and killed three American doctors and wounded an American nurse. One of the doctors had visited and worked at the hospital for seven years. The incident was like the many *green on blue* attacks that have plagued international military forces. The motives for the attack were unknown. No one, including the Taliban, has claimed responsibility. CURE Hospital is sponsored by a U.S.-based Christian charity and was founded in Kabul in 2005, the year before FMIC was formally inaugurated. Like FMIC, CURE focused on women's and children's care. I have visited the hospital and met CURE International's founder, Dr. Scott Harrison.

EPILOGUE:
ON REFLECTION

FMIC's founding partners entered their alliance for lofty purposes. Afghan children were disabled and dying with diseases and conditions for which there were no sources of treatment. Something had to be done to address that. Afghan institutions and infrastructure had been destroyed by decades of war. New institutions had to be created to train health professionals and elevate their capacity to achieve the highest standards of care. Toward these purposes, the French sought to renew historic institutional links between Afghanistan and centers of academic excellence in their country. The AKDN sought to introduce its renowned university to create a center of tertiary care, education, and research that could become the hub of a comprehensive, cross-border, integrated health system in Central Asia. Despite the partners' noble intentions and, despite FMIC's incredible success in its short history, its future is inseparable from what the future holds for the country.

Afghanistan recently conducted a presidential election, the country's first-ever democratic transfer of presidential power. At first, the election looked like an unqualified success. Surprisingly, ethnicity didn't seem to be a dominant feature in the election. The leading candidates were moderates who reached across ethnic lines to build their tickets. Over seven million voted – sixty percent of those eligible. Unfortunately, no candidate achieved more than fifty percent of total votes cast, the number required to avoid a runoff between the top two vote getters, former Foreign Minister Abdullah Abdullah and ex-Finance Minister Ashraf Ghani.

Over the next three months Afghanistan was thrown into turmoil. A runoff election was conducted. Ghani and Abdulla threw accusations of fraud back and forth. Through negotiations brokered by John Kerry, both candidates agreed to a total re-count under UN supervision and to form a unity government with a new post of *chief executive* – a position similar to that of prime minister – to be filled by the runner-up. Finally, in mid-September the candidates announced they had resolved all their differences and agreed to the conditions of a unity government. The re-count was completed and Ghani was declared the victor.

At ceremonies on September 29, 2014 Ghani was sworn in as President and, under terms of the power-sharing agreement, immediately swore Abdullah in as chief executive. At this point, many Afghans are breathing a big sigh of relief. There is hope the candidates' enormous effort of reconciliation will start the country on a path toward peace and stability. It remains to be seen whether that will happen.

After more than a decade of involvement in Afghanistan, it seems the international community may be ready to walk away from it. In the minds of many the job is finished. Osama bin Laden was long ago killed and Al-Qaida and the Taliban have been routed. Many hold the view, "We've done what we went there for. Now let's go home." Some argue that the sunk costs are too great to prematurely withdraw from the country. Too many lives have been lost and too much money has been spent. Others argue that the opportunity still exists to create a stable and secure environment and now is not the time to walk away. The stakes are too high to let Afghanistan ever again become a haven for terrorists.

In a September 12, 2014 speech at Georgetown University's Center for Security Studies, John Sopko, Washington's Special Inspector General for Afghanistan Reconstruction, said the United States has spent more than $104 billion to rebuild Afghanistan – an unprecedented amount – more money than it spent for any one country in history and more than it spent to re-build Europe after World War II. Moreover, he said the U.S. Congress has appropriated another $16 billion for reconstruction that is waiting to be spent.

Success of development and humanitarian projects in Afghanistan won't just happen because donors or sponsors throw money at them and then walk away. There is no question that corruption is rampant. Donors and project implementers have to work within that reality. Successful development outcomes require tenacity and discipline, a willingness to pay attention to detail. Somebody has to keep a close eye on the shop and monitor outcomes. These elements are not magic. They are good business practices.

In a 2011 report entitled *Evaluating Foreign Assistance to Afghanistan*, the U.S. Senate Foreign Relations Committee – chaired by then Senator John Kerry, now Secretary of State in the Obama Administration – examined closely how the United States was spending civilian aid dollars in Afghanistan. The committee report set forth three basic conditions that should be met before money is spent for development projects: they should be *necessary, achievable*, and *sustainable*. A simple rule should be followed:

"Do not implement projects if Afghans cannot sustain them. Development . . . will only succeed if Afghans are legitimate partners and there is a path toward sustainability." Those prescribed *basic conditions* seem to aptly fit FMIC. I believe FMIC is one of Afghanistan's most remarkable reconstruction success stories. In this book, I have tried to describe its success and how it so rapidly established itself as the preeminent center for extraordinary health care and health sciences learning in Afghanistan. I have identified the factors that underpin its success and set it apart from less-successful developmental ventures undertaken in the country during the past decade. In many ways, those factors are the basics of any solid and successful enterprise – a genuine and purposeful commitment by each of the sponsors, a strong sense of direction and vision with emphasis on capacity development of Afghans, good governance, sound management, and transparency.

The application of a well-crafted and well-executed public-private partnership at FMIC has provided an effective model for international partners to interact with the Afghan government and individual Afghan citizens, and to mutually explore and demonstrate the importance of moral and fiduciary principles like good governance and management, integrity, and transparency. While not a panacea, FMIC's model of public-private partnership is worth consideration by any donor, or entity interested in developing Afghanistan's civil society. Whether or not the model is replicated in kind, many of its principles of design and execution have demonstrated their merit, as evidenced through their implementation in practice.

FMIC is not yet sustainable. On the human capacity side, great progress has been made. Afghan doctors and other health professionals increasingly demonstrate the ability to independently deliver health care of the highest standard, but their numbers are still too few. More of them need continued access to advanced training and exposure to international best practices. On the financial side, FMIC does not yet offer the breadth and diversity of services to generate sufficient income from those who can afford to pay and thereby help offset the cost of caring for those who cannot. Continued support will be required for the foreseeable future.

Over the past decade, I've traveled to Afghanistan nearly sixty times. I've had the opportunity to meet and talk with Afghans of all characteristics – male and female, poor and well-off, well-educated and barely educated – Pashtun, Tajik, Hazara, and more. I've been deeply impressed with their courage and resilience, as well as their appreciation of the international community's efforts in their behalf. The men and women I've met – doctors, nurses, bureaucrats, merchants, small business owners, and farmers – all desire peace, good health, and a reasonable quality of life.

Afghans are rightfully concerned about their country's future. They fear a return to the savagery of the Mujahidin period. Dr. Jalil Wardak expresses both the fear and the hope of his countrymen. Jalil realizes that politics are always difficult to understand and, in Afghanistan, it is even more difficult. "Everything depends on security and stability. We hope our government will stabilize and the international community will not leave before finishing their goals here. With international help and by the grace of God we will have a very good future, especially for my children and for all Afghan children. I hope they will not suffer like I suffered in my last thirty years. My colleagues all think the same. Of course we have a lot of problems, but these problems will not stop us. We have good hope and visions for our future.

When we have international societies with us and partnerships like FMIC, we can have hope for the future. This hope gives me energy to go ahead."

Jalil's hope is a good place for my story to end. The fact that the FMIC partnership is a cause for his hope gives me great satisfaction. FMIC's story is just beginning. My involvement with it has truly been one of the most uplifting experiences of my life. Something has happened at FMIC that transcends mere good business practices. What accounts for that? Maybe it's the nature of the institution and what it does. Children's lives have been saved that would have otherwise been lost. Little crippled bodies have been repaired and families' lives have been improved. Maybe it's the relentless quest at FMIC to pursue excellence in whatever it does. Or maybe it's the respect for human dignity and diversity that has been instilled into FMIC's culture. A precious milieu of passion and empathy has been created. Staff, patients, and families from different walks of life, different cultures, and different religious beliefs interact with understanding, tenderness, and compassion. Whatever the cause, however it came about – FMIC is a place of miracles.

CPSIA information can be obtained
at www.ICGtesting.com
Printed in the USA
FSOW01n2027260416
19719FS